"If health is wealth, *Like A Natural Woman* is a gold mine of medical information. Ziba zeros in on traditional, non-traditional, holistic, and sacred pharmacology that will benefit readers of all ages. Each natural woman case study removes myths and misconceptions and offers sisters a wide range of modern medical options, along with ancient healing remedies."
—Dr. Gwendolyn Goldsby Grant, Psychologist, Advice Columnist, *Essence Magazine,* and author of *The Best Kind Of Loving*

"*Like A Natural Woman* offers not only topnotch traditional health advice but the latest on alternative healing. No matter what ails you, you'll find it an enjoyable, informative read. I highly recommend it."

—Valerie Wilson Wesley, author
Ain't Nobody's Business If I Do
"The Tamara Hayle Mysteries"

"That's right, sistahs! We now have a guide to alternative healing written with our particular needs and concerns front and center. From cysts and fibroids to menstrual symptoms, herbs, and reflexology, *Like A Natural Woman* gives you answers that will help you to take back your power and honor your body temple by healing the natural way.

—Debrena Jackson Gandy, author
All the Joy You Can Stand
Sacred Pampering Principles.

Like A
Natural Woman

The Black Woman's Guide to
Alternative Healing

ZIBA KASHEF

KENSINGTON PUBLISHING CORP.
http://www.kensingtonbooks.com

KENSINGTON BOOKS are published by

Kensington Publishing Corp.
850 Third Avenue
New York, NY 10022

All Kensington titles, imprints and distributed lines are available at special quantity discounts for bulk purchases for sales promotion, premiums, fund raising, educational or institutional use.

Special book excerpts or customized printings can also be created to fit specific needs. For details, write or phone the office of the Kensington Special Sales Manager: Kensington Publishing Corp., 850 Third Avenue, New York, NY 10022, Attn. Special Sales Department. Phone: 1-800-221-2647.

Library of Congress Card Catalogue Number: 00-103526
ISBN 1-57566-630-8

First Printing: January 2001
10 9 8 7 6 5 4 3 2 1

Printed in the United States of America

Contents

Contents

Foreword by
Marcellus Walker, MD, LAc

It seems that at no other time in history has so much been asked of the African-American woman. This is because life is moving so fast, the amount of responsibilities has increased, but the time to complete them remains the same. With all this activity, some things frequently get neglected. This may be a contributing factor to the health problems that African Americans are experiencing at epidemic levels. Our health crisis hits African-American women especially hard. It reflects the fact that our personal and health needs are falling by the wayside.

The process of self-forgetting and self-neglect may be subtle. It can show up as a symptom of searching for something outside of ourselves. We may try relationships, activities, clothes or food, but nothing quite fills the space. At some point we may choose to stop and consider that the missing "peace" may be a deeper, richer relationship with ourselves. The question is: *How do I do that? How do I achieve this deeper relationship, and how much time will it take? What will I look like when I get there? Will my friends be the same? Can I do it?* All of these questions are natural, and making the choice to deepen the relationship with yourself may be the single most important factor in your health.

To remember ourselves we must first understand the broader picture of how health and disease take place. We need to understand what our needs are and on what level these needs are manifested.

In order to do this, we have to begin with the principle: understanding that within our overall system we are made up of levels. Each level has its own needs. We have a physical level, which has been the focus of conventional medicine. Examples of our needs on this level include rest and sleep, proper food and nutrition, clean water and air, and vitamins and minerals.

In addition, we also have an organized energy level. We know this intuitively since we talk about our energy all the time. One of the most common things that patients say to me is: "I wish I had more energy," or "I don't know where my energy has gone." In fact, we have an entire energy structure, which if out of balance, can lead to physical, emotional, or mental issues. Many of the alternative or natural therapies are medications for this level of our system. This is why *Like a Natural Woman,* and the approaches that are talked about in it, are so important. Conventional medications just don't treat this level.

The other levels that make up our system are not real levels per se but areas of need. We have emotional needs, mental needs, and spiritual needs. If these needs are not addressed for ourselves with quality time, they can stress our overall system and eventually lead to physical problems. Therefore, to achieve optimal health we need to achieve balance within ourselves by giving balance to the various levels or needs. This can only be achieved by adding natural healing methods to our conventional medical approaches, for the best results and optimum health.

The key to recouping our health is to take a broader view of what health is. Our ancestors have always held this broader view of health and healing. Therefore, it should come naturally to us since we depended on natural or alternative approaches to manage our health at a time when we had no other choices. We also looked into these areas for our solace and for hope. Our ancestors were right all along. Grounding our health in natural approaches is a good foundation, indeed. We also need to use what works from conventional approaches when appropriate.

In the end, it is all about balance. We need to balance our individual needs with those around us. We need to take care of ourselves on more than one level, and we need to continue to do so throughout our lives and as things change. This is why *Like a Natural Woman* is such an important work; it will help you better understand the levels of your system and give you a clue as to how to navigate within these spaces. I wish you the best in your journey; I know that you can do it. Just remember not to judge yourself, never abandon yourself, and spend more time listening to yourself. Each step is a learning experience that allows you to be the natural woman that you are.

Marcellus Walker, MD, LAc
Founder, africanamericanhealth.com
Coauthor, *Natural Health for African Americans*

Acknowledgments

I give thanks:

First and foremost, to God be all the glory.

To the women who have allowed me to share their stories of healing in order to help others.

To all the healers who contributed their ideas and expertise to this work and to all of the healers who are changing the way the world looks at health and healing. Special thanks to Dr. Marcellus A. Walker, MD, LAc for reading the manuscript and serving as advisor.

To the researchers who contributed their time and talent: Zurn Porter, Patricia Mason Woods, Rachel Christmas Derrick, Kendra Lee, Michelle Longo, Teresa Ridley, Regina Cash, Pittershawn Palmer, April McKoy.

To my agent Barbara Lowenstein, editor Karen Thomas, Janice Rossi, and the staff at Kensington Publishing for working to bring an important idea to fruition.

Acknowledgments

To the team at *Essence* for supporting me and this project: Susan L. Taylor, Monique Greenwood, Robin Stone, LaVon Leak-Wilks, and all the editors.

For cheering me on: Linda Villarosa, Rosemarie Robotham, Joan Morgan-Murray, Marisol Booth, Olivia Smith, Tamala Edwards.

To Tony Johnston, for your gentle spirit and open heart.

To my family, for your unconditional love.

Like A
Natural Woman

Chapter 1

~

Livin' Healthy

NATURAL WOMAN: JACKIE LEWIS

When Jackie Lewis was about 44 years old, she started waking up in the middle of the night, her heart racing. She went to the doctor, who told her that her thyroid, triggered by the changes of peri-menopause, was acting irregularly. He recommended surgery on her thyroid, but Jackie, then a New York City boutique owner, re-sisted and decided instead to change her life. "I asked for them to give me time," says Jackie. "I was not interested in an operation." She took that time to take stock of her lifestyle.

"My life had been to go out at night and have drinks and party and eat," she explains. "But I recognized it was killing me. Here it was affecting my body."

Jackie had heard about a book called Heal Your Body *(Hay House, Inc.) by metaphysical teacher Louise L. Hay, which purports that all physical illness has an emotional cause. After reading the book, she began repeating an affirmation that, according to Hay, corresponded to the thyroid:* I move beyond old limitations and now allow myself to express freely and creatively. *That was the first step in her healing. Following her instinct to completely transform her life, she also fasted on juices for two weeks and underwent a series of ten colonic hydrotherapy treatments. She stopped eating meat and drinking alcohol. Though Jackie had initially taken medication to manage her overactive thyroid, she weaned herself off of it as she embraced a new lifestyle. "In six months, my thyroid had healed," she explains.*

During this healing period, Jackie also started practicing yoga and learning about the value of deep breathing. "I know I was alive, but I wasn't breathing," *she says. Like most of us, Jackie realized she was only taking in small breaths instead of breathing from the belly. "When you are breathing, it's almost as if you have direct connection to the higher powers, or whatever you call that energy," she notes. "Once you breathe, your life changes."*

Jackie now sees her health challenge as a wake-up call. The call was soon followed by her decision to leave the fashion business and pursue her dream of opening a holistic spa in Jamaica. Though she didn't know exactly what a "holistic spa" was at the time, she listened to the inner voice that told her to pitch a tent on a reef in Negril and allow her dream to unfold. Gradually, her spa on the reef developed into a unique facility that offers clients everything from yoga and light island cuisine to emotional healing retreats. As the owner of Jackie's on the Reef, Jackie has gained insight not only into her own transformation but into the need for healing in others. "Black women call and say they want to come and the first thing they do is go to the beach and party," she says about many of her clients. "It's has to do with our consciousness. We feel guilty about pampering ourselves." Jackie believes the self-neglect goes back to our history and our vision of ourselves as black women. "I question what we think about ourselves. For so many years and generations, the black woman has been nurturing everyone—the family and other people's children," she notes. "We don't know what it is to take care of ourselves."

Healthy Living: Caring for Ourselves

Jackie Lewis's formerly stressful lifestyle left her vulnerable to an illness that forced her to let go of her unhealthy routine and heed her mind and body's pleas. Her experience is not unusual. Because black women are often working demanding jobs and in many cases also raising kids and catering to mates, elderly relatives, and the community, we neglect to take good care of ourselves. At the end of the day, we have little energy left to tune in to our own needs, let alone respond to them. It's no surprise Superwoman gets sick and sicker than most.

One of the most difficult challenges that sisters face is putting ourselves—and our health—first. Taking care of ourselves sounds simple enough, but it's not. With our multiple responsibilities and strong sense of obligation to being the backbone of our families and communities, we all too often shelve our needs and think life is supposed to be that way. Over time, self-denial and self-sacrifice form the basis for our identities and our lifestyle decisions: *"I'm too busy to slow down." "I don't have time for exercise." "I can't afford to take a break."* "We tend to take care of everybody else," says Ruby Carroll Simpkins, MD, a California physician whose practice offers alternative therapies such as massage, acupuncture, and biofeedback. "But if you're not at your best, you can't be your best for anyone else."

Taking care of ourselves means taking off the Superwoman cape, says Dr. Maisha Tianuru, ND, MT, of the Afrikan Center of Well Being in Houston. "We can have it all, just maybe not all at the same time," Tianuru notes. "I tell my patients, 'Please include yourself in the process of life *first*. You cannot give what you don't have.' "

Are you taking the very best care of yourself? If not, it's time to put your health back on your list of priorities. Good health is our greatest resource; without it, we can't do all that we want to do. "Good health is a way to prepare yourself for better opportunities," says Camille Finley, personal trainer and host of *Shape Up Chicago,* including that promotion or new project. To tap in to the powers of natural healing, we must first choose a more balanced lifestyle.

Living in Balance

Natural healers believe that good health is more than the absence of disease; it's a balance of mental, physical, emotional, and spiritual well-being. If any part of our whole selves is lacking or out of balance, a health challenge--a nagging ache, a distracting feeling of dis-ease or anxiety, fatigue, or pain—may result. Those distress signals are the body's cries for help that we, as black women, too often ignore because we're accustomed to focusing our energies and efforts outside of ourselves. Living in balance means listening to—and attending to—the needs of the body, mind, and spirit continually.

Our ancestors understood the meaning of balance, and its connection to well-being. In his book *The Healing Wisdom of Africa* (J. P. Tarcher), West African shaman Malidoma Patrice Somé writes, "Methods of healing must take into account the energetic or spiritual condition that is in turmoil, thereby affecting the physical condition. If you focus only on the physical translation of the underlying energetic disorder, then you are ignoring the source of the physical illness." He adds, "If you instead address the energy of the mind and spirit, whose status is affecting the physical body, then you are likely to heal truly."

But like eating a "balanced diet," living a balanced life is easier to imagine than to do. Even those of us who eat heathily and exercise regularly may occasionally engage in other self-defeating behaviors. A vegetarian who doesn't sleep isn't healthy. An athlete who lives with anger isn't truly fit and whole. A teetotaler who never takes a break or a vacation isn't well, or as well as she could be.

Assessing Ourselves

It often takes a health challenge to get folks to pay attention to their body, mind, and spirit, to stop and notice that more sleep or more water or more relaxation is required. A better way is to get in the habit of tuning in to the messages our mind-body-spirit system sends us before a problem strikes. When was the last time someone asked, "How are you?" and you answered the question truthfully? Every day, look in the mirror and ask, *How are you?* Say the words out loud and listen for a response. Take this opportunity right now to write down the answer in terms of your total well-being. Don't think, censor, or revise; just feel and then write:

Self-Awareness Tool 1

How Are You?

_____

_____

_____

_____

_____

_____

_____

_____

Writing down or saying how you feel simply brings that sense of your well-being—or lack thereof—to your awareness. When we are feeling good, we can enjoy it; when we are not, we can respond to the need or needs at hand. This checking in with ourselves helps us stay in balance. Without the awareness, however, we lose touch with ourselves and our health often suffers.

In addition to awareness, balanced living relies on the habits we adopt and sustain day in and day out. Even if you are taking generally good care of yourself, it's easy to lose track of how often you eat on a busy day or how many hours you sleep, for example. But the ways in which we conduct our lives either support our body's natural healing ability or undermine it. Are your habits helping—or hurting?

Self-Awareness Tool 2

Lifestyle Habits Quiz

Place a check by each statement that is true for you.

____ I eat *at least* three balanced meals, each including a vegetable or fruit, each day.

____ I drink six to eight eight-ounce glasses of pure water each day.

____ I take a multivitamin/multimineral supplement each day.

____ I enjoy some type of physical activity (walking, gardening, yoga) for *at least* thirty minutes each day, or on most days.

____ I spend at least ten minutes of quiet time alone (meditating, praying, deep breathing, daydreaming) each day.

____ I do something to work toward fulfilling my dreams—read about starting a business, practice an instrument, indulge in a hobby like quilting—each day or each week.

____ I spend at least fifteen minutes outdoors in sunlight each day.

____ I take steps to minimize stress (take breaks, call a supportive friend) each day.

____ I avoid smoking and secondhand cigarette smoke.

____ I drink no more than one to three alcoholic beverages per week.

____ I avoid caffeinated coffee, tea, and colas.

____ I get approximately seven hours sleep per night.

If you were able to check off most or all of the items, you are probably already living a basically balanced lifestyle and practicing good health. If you only checked a few, however, think about why and whether you might want to make a change in one area or another. The point of the quiz is to not to chastise yourself or feel guilty but to help you evaluate your lifestyle and habits in order to affirm or change them. You can also return to this list to periodically to check your progress.

Check Your Checkups

The number of sisters getting screened for common infections and illnesses has increased significantly in recent years, but too many of us still miss lifesaving tests. Eighty-four percent of all African-American women aged 18 and older got their Pap tests in 1994, an increase from 68 percent in 1987. Thirty-seven percent of all black women over 50 reported that they did not get a mammogram within the last two years in 1994, and 25 percent said they did not have a clinical breast exam in that time. More than a third of pregnant black women do not begin prenatal care in the first trimester, which may contribute to our higher rates of premature delivery, low birthweight, and infant mortality.

If you have not already seen your main health care provider for a physical, your obstetrician-gynecologist for a pelvic exam, as well as your dentist and eye care professionals within the last twelve months, make these appointments now. Don't wait for a health problem to occur to go to the doctor. Regular checkups and testing can help detect problems early and prevent disease. Delayed exams lead to delayed diagnoses and unnecessary concern and suffering.

Tests to Take

Test	Tests for	Age to Start	How Often
Physical exam	Vital signs	Birth	Every two years or more often (ask your provider)
	Height/weight		
	Ears, eyes, throat		
	Respiration		
	Pulse		
	Blood pressure		
	Blood tests*		
	Urinalysis**		
Pelvic exam	Infections, growths Vagina, ovary, uterus	18, or younger if sexually active	Annually
Pap smear	Abnormal cervical cells Sexually transmitted infections	18, or younger if sexually active	Annually
Clinical breast exam	Lumps, discharge	18	Annually
Mammogram	Abnormal cells, lumps	35 for first x-ray	Annually after 40
HIV	Virus that causes AIDS	18 or younger if at risk (ask provider)	
Dental	Cavities, infections	Before 1	Every 6 months
Eye	Vision, glaucoma	Before 1	Annually

*Blood tests check complete blood count and screen for anemia, cholesterol, diabetes, and infections, among other health problems.

**Urinalysis screens for infections and abnormal function of kidney and liver among other health indicators.

Stress: Killing Us Softly?

We know that emotional stress is a part of living. But excessive stress may be the greatest threat to a balanced life and to your healing. Why is stress dangerous? Our bodies' built-in fight-or-flight response is designed to protect us from harm and ready us to handle life's challenges—a sudden death, loss of a job, a life-threatening illness. In this sense, stress is our friend. But when stress is ongoing or chronic, it becomes a poison. The constant flux of stress hormones such as adrenalin and cortisol can overwhelm our mind-body systems, sapping the body's ability to fend for itself. Chronic negative stress weakens our immune systems by diminishing the production of white blood cells—some of the body's most powerful warriors against disease. That's why an anxiety-producing job, relationship, or financial problem can literally be hazardous to our health. Today folks visit their doctors more often because of stress-related health problems—such as upper respiratory infections, allergies, migraines, ulcers, high blood pressure, and depression—than any other.

As career women, mothers, and family and community leaders, black women live with extraordinarily high levels of stress. Pressure-filled lives combined with the anxiety of coping with sexism *and* racism leave us particularly vulnerable to the ravages of stress. A 1997 Duke University Medical Center study revealed that when thirty healthy African-American women were provoked by racially charged comments in debates with white researchers, they experienced sharp and prolonged increases in their heart rates and blood pressures. This strong reaction did not occur when the women debated another provocative but nonracial topic. Just imagine how often our minds and bodies are assaulted in this way in real life without anyone taking notice or measuring the impact! The chronic stress of dealing with discrimination on a daily basis has unknown effects but, the Duke researchers concluded, may contribute to higher rates of hypertension and heart disease among black people.

To make matters worse, as "strong black women," we are not accustomed to—and we have often not allowed ourselves to—incor-

9

porating stress-reducing activities and strategies into our lives. Besides prayer and reliance on our informal and formal sister circles, there is little tradition of stress prevention or management in our community. We have only begun to experiment with powerful natural healing tools such as meditation, massage, exercise, and therapy. Less healthy but common coping mechanisms like overeating and smoking only compound the negative effects of stress, leading to health problems such as weight gain, obesity, cancer, and heart disease.

Being "stressed out" often or all the time can kill. In 1998, The Rockefeller University scientists reported that the ongoing emotional stress that begins in our heads can lead to real changes in our bodies, including suppressed immunity, muscle weakening, bone loss, memory loss, increased insulin levels, abdominal fat, and atherosclerosis, or hardening of the arteries. Over time, these changes set the stage for long-term health problems. For example, a suppressed immune system can make us vulnerable to everything from colds to cancer. High insulin levels and abdominal fat are a recipe for diabetes. Atherosclerosis is a step on the road to a heart attack.

Though stress is ever present, the good news is we are always in control of the way we deal with it. We can draw upon multiple natural healing tools to minimize the sources of stress in our lives before they result in *distress*. The first step, again, is awareness. "Our bodies are actually barometers, signaling all the time when we're under stress," says naturopath Tianuru. "So it's real important to be aware, to read the barometer and use that information. That is your first step in alleviating the actual stress. Say, 'I'm under stress. I'm aware of that. What can I do about it?' "

According to Tianuru, signs of mental and emotional stress include forgetfulness, inability to concentrate, errors in judgment or distance, distorted perceptions, worry, irritability, suspicion, feelings of worthlessness, self-criticism, withdrawal, crying, and isolation. The physical manifestations might include increased heart rate, tightness in the chest, sweaty palms, ticks, twitching, teeth grinding, diarrhea, vomiting, overeating, headaches, skin eruptions, irritable bowel syndrome, chronic fatigue syndrome, and more. (If you have symptoms, see your health-care provider to rule out other causes.)

Take a few minutes to identify the causes of ongoing stress in your life. What are you worried about? In what areas of your life are you most troubled—relationships, work, health, or family? Write your top five answers down on the following lines. Then next to each stress source, jot down an ideal solution:

Source of Stress   **Ideal Solution**

_____   _____

_____   _____

_____   _____

_____   _____

_____   _____

Even if the solution seems impossible, write it down anyway. As long as it is a positive solution, you can work toward achieving it by breaking it down into small, practical steps. The very act of writing the cause of your stress down gives it less power to run your life—and wear down your health.

To combat stress, Tianuru suggests two surefire strategies:

- Breathe! Stop whatever you are doing and inhale deeply from the diaphragm. Take six deep, cleansing breaths. This will cause your blood pressure to immediately drop. Whatever the situation, remember to smile and breathe.
- Walk your walk. The simple act of putting one foot in front of the other gets oxygen flowing in even the most stressed-out body. It's gentle and it's free.

The gentle exercise routines described below and meditation are additional ways to de-stress. Finding the stress solution or solutions that work for you and committing to them regularly may be the most important lifestyle change and natural health-promoting step you ever make.

Another antidote to stress is the simple yet powerful serenity prayer we are all familiar with. I keep a copy of it posted above my desk at work.

God grant me the serenity
to accept the things I cannot change,
the courage to change the things I can,
and the wisdom to know the difference.

Exercise as Natural Medicine

In addition to making us feel energized and helping us reach and maintain a healthy weight, physical activity has a surprising number of health benefits. Research is showing that exercise is good for our bodies and spirits. Regular physical activity improves circulation and lowers blood pressure, helps us maintain muscle and bone strength, slows aging, relieves the symptoms of depression and anxiety, and helps us get more restful sleep.

More and more black women are participating in sports and fitness programs these days in walking groups, exercise classes, and African dance studios. Yet too many sisters do not get any physical activity during the day. According to a 1992 Centers for Disease Control and Prevention survey, 43 percent of African-American women ages 18 and older participated in no "leisure-time physical activity." Studies have shown that some blacks tend to think of exercise as a source of stress rather than as a way of alleviating it. With all of the responsibilities we bear, exercise—especially as it is defined by the mainstream culture as "no pain, no gain"—may seem more of a torturous chore than a source of pleasure and well-being. But the lack of physical activity, however we define it, is a major risk factor for disease, nearly as detrimental as smoking.

Whether you currently exercise or not, alternatives to conventional forms of exercise engage the spirit and emotions as well as the body. Eastern practices such as yoga, tai chi, and chi kung tone and strengthen the body while also offering ways to ease stress, improve concentration, and grow spiritually. African-derived practices such as capoeira challenge us physically while also connecting us with our cultural roots and community. If you are already doing a sport, taking aerobics classes, or walking, you can complement your routine with one of these more holistic "workouts." If you have not exercised in a while and are turned off by the idea of going to a gym or by exercise in general, you may be delighted by how the following alternatives can help you experience your body in a new and profound way.

Yoga

Though yoga originated in the East, images in Egyptian temples depict Africans in positions strikingly similar to yoga positions. This ancient Hindu discipline is as much a spiritual path as a physical practice. Meaning "union," the word "yoga" is usually used to describe a series of postures (asanas) and breathing exercises (pranayama).Yoga has endless natural health benefits. Beyond the obvious benefit of making your muscles and joints more flexible, yoga can also help tone muscles throughout the body; improve balance and coordination; stimulate respiration, circulation, and digestion; boost energy; and even relieve menstrual problems!

The most important benefit may simply be that yoga focuses your awareness. "You train your mind to stay on what you are doing and that carries over into your life," says Vivinne Williams, owner of Sattva Yoga and Wellness in New York City. That heightened awareness can help with weight loss, flexibility, back problems, and even high blood pressure, Williams notes.

The form of yoga practiced in the West is known as hatha yoga, yoga of body and mind, but there are many different styles of hatha yoga that range from gentle, slow-paced regimens to ones that are as challenging as any aerobics class. In an ashtanga or power yoga class, students perform yoga postures quickly enough to work up a sweat. Iyengar yoga focuses more on perfecting body alignment and hold-

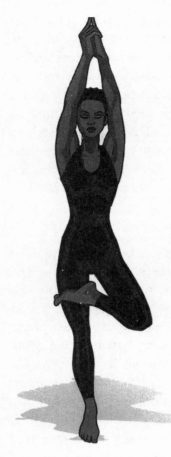

Yoga
This Hatha Yoga posture, known as the Tree, is just one of a series of postures that, combined with breathing techniques, brings balance and unity to the body and mind.

ing the postures for several minutes. "The tradition I teach at Kripalu is more centered on the heart and emotional growth," says Williams. She suggests taking a couple of beginner classes at local yoga schools to find something you like.

Tai chi

Though tai chi is a centuries-old martial art, the way it is practiced today is anything but combative. This physical, mental, and spiritual regimen is based on the Chinese notion of releasing and generating *qi* (pronounced "chi") or life force energy, and creating harmony in the body and with nature. The series of basic moves and stances are performed in a graceful dance. Each move, which involves *yin* (yielding) and *yang* (thrusting) phases, is done in rhythm with your inhalation and exhalation. In addition to releasing tension throughout the body, through tai chi you can improve balance, flexibility, concentration, and the functioning of many organ systems and the immune system. In studies, tai chi has been shown to naturally lower blood pressure. The underlying purpose of relieving tension and increasing energy flow can help in managing stress. You can practice tai chi in groups, with a partner, or alone and for as little as ten minutes a day to feel better, more balanced, relaxed and healthy.

Chi kung (qigong)

Meaning energy *(qi)* work *(gong)* or working with life energy, chi kung is the practice of controlling and directing the flow of life force throughout the body. This harmonizes the mind-body system while enhancing health. To unblock stagnant life energy, practitioners of active chi kung learn correct posture and a variety of graceful exercises; passive or tranquil chi kung includes breathing techniques, visualization, and concentration. The chi kung program not only boosts energy, but increases physical strength, speeds metabolism and digestion, and improves sleep. It can also increase the chance of recovery from serious illness like cancer when used in conjunction with Western medicine. Practicing chi kung for twenty minutes or more a day can reduce stress and increase inner peace.

Pilates

Developed by a German physical trainer named Joseph H. Pilates, the Pilates Method of Body Conditioning is the "science and art of coordinated body-mind-spirit development through natural movements under strict control of will." Popular with dancers and athletes, pilates is based on six principles: concentration, control, centering, movement quality, precision and breathing. Pilates devotees perform a series of over sixty core exercises, many of which require special tools and equipment. Doing pilates for as little as ten minutes a day, four times a week can help you improve posture, muscle tone, and flexibility and enhance immune function. By developing balance and self-control, practitioners also enjoy a boost in confidence.

Capoeira

An Angolan martial art that was transported to Brazil by enslaved Africans, capoeira is a form of self-defense that can also bring balance and discipline to the body and mind. Capoeiristas learn defensive moves on their own, then practice them with a partner in a graceful dance. Pairs take turns as the class, gathered together in a circle, watches and chants to the beat of drums. Students of capoeira build strength and increase agility. Being on the alert for an attack move also improves mental concentration.

African Dance

Set to an ancestral beat that our bodies understand intuitively, African dance is truly a spiritual workout as well as a physical and mental one. The various styles of African dance—barambaye, lamban, odunde—are not just dances, but expressions or celebrations. With its emphasis on joyful expression and movement, African dance encourages us to let go and respond to a natural rhythm. The vibrant, loosely coordinated movements work our hearts and muscles, boost energy, and help us develop discipline. The beat, the loose-fitting African attire, and the relationship to the drummer reconnect us with our heritage.

How Much Is Enough?

If you're among those sisters who exercise at least thirty minutes per session, most days of the week, keep it up. If not, it's time to decide how you will fit regular physical activity into your life. There are many ways to get your body moving that are enjoyable and fun. If time is an issue, don't give up. Researchers now say that effective exercise can be accumulated throughout the day, and can include moderate activities such as walking instead of driving short distances, gardening, or playing with your kids. In other words, it all counts and it's all good.

Regardless of how you choose to exercise, it's key to make the time and to do it consistently. If you consider how you spend your time each day, thirty minutes is not unreasonable and your body is worth it. Check with your health care provider first if you are over age 40 and have not exercised in a while, or if you have a chronic disease (heart disease, diabetes, hypertension, arthritis). For motivation, ask a fitness-minded sistafriend, mate, or relative to join you.

Once you've picked an aerobic activity you enjoy, add strength training and stretching for flexibility. You can lift free weights or do calisthenics such as push-ups and sit-ups two or three days a week. Building muscle strength will give you a toned figure, help you burn calories more efficiently and prevent injury. To flex your flexibility, stretch regularly. This will keep muscles and joints limber. One of the many exercise books and tapes on the market, fitness magazines, or a certified personal trainer can help you devise a program that fits in to your life. Additional fitness tips:

- Remember to always warm up for two to five minutes before vigorous exercise to warm the muscles and loosen ligaments. Do light stretching of major muscle groups to avoid injury. Also cool down and stretch after exercise to lessen muscle soreness.
- Know your "target heart zone." Grab a calculator and subtract your age from 220 to get your maximum heart rate (MHR). Multiply that number by .65 and then .80. The two numbers give you your target heart zone range.
- Take your pulse. During exercise, count pulse beats on your wrist or neck for 15 seconds; multiply by 4. It should be in your target heart zone.
- Every month or so increase either the duration, intensity, or frequency of the activities you enjoy most often.

- Set goals—miles run, pounds lost, pounds lifted—and reward yourself when you meet them.
- Drink water before, during, and after workouts to replenish lost fluids and keep the body cool.
- Invest in the appropriate shoes, sports bras, and other equipment you need to avoid discomfort and injury.

Many people start exercise programs but fewer keep them going. There are many reasons—and many more excuses—for putting exercise off: lack of time, money, motivation, accessible facilities, support from family and friends. But if we stop exercising, the benefits diminish within just a couple of weeks and completely disappear within a few months. If you stop exercising for any reason, forgive yourself and start again. It's not about rules, but fun and feeling good. "Make the program yours," says Finley. "If you're tired, just do ten minutes and be okay with that. After you take ownership and realize that there are no rules, you start to relax and incorporate more things as time goes on. It takes time to make it consistent and make it a part of your life."

Making Good Health a Habit

Ten Natural Health Habits for Every Day

1. Drink a glass of water every two hours. This should add up to at least eight glasses by the end of the day. Our bodies don't immediately signal us that we are dehydrated, so we need to replenish lost fluids before we feel thirsty. Lack of water can undermine our health and cause fatigue, among other problems. To get in the habit, drink water first thing in the morning, with each meal, and before going to bed at night. Choose bottled spring water or filtered drinking water to protect your body from contaminants.

2. Experience nature. Visit a park or beach. Tianuru, who says she feels unsettled if she hasn't touched nature during the day, suggests

starting a garden. Being in nature and in contact with natural things has tremendous healing power. The natural light you receive also gives your body important nutrients including vitamin D, which may be lacking in people of color. Sunlight is also a natural mood booster.

3. Check your thoughts. Our thoughts create our life experiences, including our health experience. Many negative thoughts run through our minds each day without our even noticing. Just as you learn to be aware of the foods you put in your body, tune in to the thoughts you allow to echo in your mind. Catch a negative thought, write it down, and create an affirmation as its opposite.

4. Reach out. Pick up the phone to call a relative or an old friend. Creating and sustaining positive relationships in our lives are important for our well-being. After you call your loved one, consider also reconciling with someone from whom you are estranged.

5. Laugh and play. They say laughter is good medicine and it is because it reconnects us with the natural joy of life. If you can't find inspiration, read a comic strip or watch a funny TV program or movie.

6. Praise yourself. Ever notice how good a compliment feels? Why not give it to yourself? Self-praise is fuel for high self-esteem. "If the only words of praise that you get during the day are from nobody, give them to yourself," says Tianuru. Learn to appreciate yourself as a woman and a descendent of people of greatness and honor.

7. Practice TFM (time for me). Centering yourself in solitude helps you to reenter the world stronger. "I'll tell women or suggest if you got to go close yourself up in the bathroom and sit on the toilet for five minutes, do it," says Tianuru. "Teach the kids, 'When mommy is in the bathroom for five minutes, go find something to do. Don't disturb me.' You've got to schedule yourself into life first."

8. Bring yourself joy. Cultivate your hobbies and talents. "Take an art class or a music class. Practice a hobby that you always loved to do," recommends Tianuru.

9. Go to bed on time. Individual needs vary, but if you get less than seven to eight hours of sleep at night, you may be sleep deprived. Lack of sleep can make you less alert and effective during the day, and even result in accidents. If you have a sleep disorder like insomnia, see your health care provider. Get the TV out of the bedroom

and make your environment more soothing with candles, soft colors, and music.

10. Connect with Spirit/God/your Higher Power. Spirituality has health benefits that scientists are just beginning to understand. Make a point of reconnecting with that energy first thing in the morning or last thing at night even if only for a brief reading of scripture, a prayer or conversation.

Claim Your Healthy Intentions

You may have picked up this book because you wanted to learn more about what you can do to naturally maximize your well-being, or prevent or treat a particular health problem or disease. Whatever the reason, identifying your health goals is a key step in reaching them. Take a few minutes to think about and clarify what you want in terms of your well-being. Examples might include "eat a healthier diet," "cure my fibroids," "lower my blood pressure," "lose weight," or "live a more peaceful life." Jot down up to five health goals on the following lines.

_____

_____

_____

_____

_____

Now look over your list and turn each goal into a positive affirmation. For example, instead of "I want to eat a healthier diet," write "I eat a natural, balanced, nutritious diet because it makes me feel good," or "I create good health in my life each day." The intention coupled with action puts the power to heal in your hands.

Family Health History

We share skin color, eye shape, and hair texture with our relatives. But we also may share a genetic tendency to develop specific conditions such as sickle cell disease or certain cancers. News of—or suspicion of—serious disease in black families is often met with denial and secrecy. But what we don't know can hurt us. So investigate your family health history to identify your health risks. At your next family gathering or earlier, begin to ask questions about your parents' and grandparents' health status. Do living relatives have high blood pressure, diabetes, fibroids, or lupus? What did deceased relatives die of and at what age? If family members are reluctant to talk, explain that you are collecting information that will help them and their descendents. You may need to contact distant relatives by letter or e-mail. If information is unknown, you may also need to research health records and death certificates.

Once you finish your research, use the facts you gather to evaluate your family's health. Look for any clusters of illness. If the same disease is present among first-degree relatives—mother, father, sister, brother, daughter, son—the likelihood of genetic causes increases. But don't fret: Heredity does not equal destiny; it only indicates a tendency and gives us information we can use to avoid disease and take better care of ourselves. Keep these facts in your records and share it with your health care provider.

Resources

Africanamericanhealth.com, 220 East 26th St., Suite. 1B, New York, NY 10010; (888) 313-3103; *www.africanamericanhealth.com*

American Association of Naturopathic Physicians, 601 Valley Street, Suite 105, Seattle, WA 98109, *www.naturopathic.org*

The American Yoga Association, PO Box 19986, Sarasota, FL 34276.

The Mind/Body Medical Institute, Beth Israel Deaconess Medical Center, 110 Francis St., Suite. 1A, Boston, MA 02215, *www.mindbody. harvard.edu.*

QiGong Institute, East West Academy of Healing Arts, 450 Sutter Place, Suite 2104, San Francisco, CA 94108.

Taoist T'ai Chi Society of the USA, 1060 Bannock Street, Denver, CO 80204.

8 Weeks to Optimum Health, by Andrew Weil, MD (Fawcett).

The Healing Handbook: A Beginner's Guide and Journal to Meditation, by Jodi Levy (Pocket Books).

Healthy Habits: 20 Simple Ways to Improve Your Health, by David and Anne Frahm (Putnam Publishing Group).

Heal Your Body, by Louise L. Hay (Hay House).

The Physician's Guide: Natural Health for African Americans, by Marcellus A. Walker, MD, and Kenneth B. Singleton, MD (Warner).

A Path to Healing: A Guide to Wellness for Body, Mind and Soul, by Dr. Andrea D. Sullivan (Doubleday).

Staying Strong: Reclaiming the Wisdom of African-American Healing, by Sara Lomax Reese (Editor), Kirk Johnson (Editor), Therman Evans (Editor) (William Morrow & Co.).

Chapter 2

⌖

Eating Right and Light

NATURAL WOMAN: AUDREY JACKSON

At age 38, Audrey Jackson suffered what she thought was a bad case of indigestion. In her doctor's office, she learned, however, that her chest pains were actually signs of a mild heart attack. "He told me I would not live to see 40," she recalls. At 236 pounds, Audrey could not make it up a flight of stairs without difficulty. And she already had asthma, high blood pressure, and a blood sugar level that bordered on diabetic. Her doctor's frightening prognosis forced her to make some changes. After visiting a nutritionist, Audrey began keeping a diary of her food intake as well as her mood to uncover patterns of emotional eating. She adjusted her diet to include several servings of vegetables, fruits, and grains, fish, and lots of water. She also started walking after work and joined a gym. Within ten months, she dropped more than 100 pounds.

In the years since then, Audrey has continued to shift toward a leaner, semivegetarian diet including fish, beans, and nuts for protein. She jogs or bikes most days of the week to maintain her fitness level and dives into new sports such as horseback riding and jet-

skiing. The chronic conditions she once lived with are all under control. "I have not had an asthma attack since 1994," she says emphatically. "My blood pressure is 90 over 60. No diabetes."

Let Food Be Your Medicine

Healthy eating is good medicine. The foods we eat can give us energy, help our bodies absorb key vitamins and minerals, and protect us from toxins that trigger disease. Or they can cause fatigue, slow digestion, and set the stage for weight gain, diabetes, heart disease, and other health problems that are so common among black women. According to the National Cancer Institute, eight out of ten cancers have a diet component; African-Americans have higher cancer rates than any other racial or ethnic group.

Though eating habits vary in our culture, the diets of many black women are too high in fat, cholesterol, sugar, and salt, and far too low in complex carbohydrates and fiber-rich foods. A 1997 Centers for Disease Control and Prevention survey showed that less than one in four black female high school students ate the recommended five servings of fruits and vegetables a day, and we know the habits we develop in our youth often determine our habits for life. Even those of us who make conscious efforts to learn about nutrition and eat right may not know enough about the foods we eat—and what our distinctive African body types require—to keep our bodies in their naturally healthy, disease-free state.

So how should *you* eat? There is no one answer to that question that will suit each of us individually. It depends on many factors including our individual family history, health status, preferences and belief system. But we can gather some clues from knowing what our ancestors ate and what researchers are finding out about the relationship between food and health.

Eating What Our Ancestors Ate

Why look at our ancestors diet? First to get clear on who we are. "One of the things that black women will say is, 'We're stressed out, so we have hypertension. This is part of who we are. It's a part of our heritage,' " says Saeeda Hafiz, a holistic health educator in Philadelphia. But you have to look beyond three, four, or five generations here in the United States and ask, is it of the heritage of Africans to suffer these same conditions?" In fact, our Africans ancestors had low rates of hypertension and heart disease, two health problems that are rampant in the black community. So what runs in our race is not disease, says Hafiz, but habits that have been passed down.

Not all of our African ancestors ate the same foods, of course, but research on African diets can help us draw some conclusions about what they may have survived and thrived on. Our ancestors were hunters and gatherers. According to *Funa, Food from Africa* by Renata Coetzee, foods that were indigenous to Africa and part of the traditional African diet include grains such as millet, fruits like melons, vegetables like wild spinach, and legumes such as cowpea (cousin of the black-eyed pea) and jugobean. While several kinds of insects and some wild game, fish, and shellfish were also eaten, meat was considered "only a visitor" in the diet, and milk was served soley to babies or to the elderly or infirm. With its high-fiber, low-fat content "the traditional diet was therefore nutritious by modern standards," Coetzee writes.

In *The Africa Cookbook: Tastes of the Continent,* author Jessica B. Harris makes the point that little is known about the health benefits of the traditional African diet because so little is still known about Africa. In fact, Harris notes, African food is not only nutritious fare that has inspired cooks around the world, but is likely a progenitor of the much-touted Mediterranean diet. "As in the Mediterranean diet, meat is not the centerpiece of the plate but rather a taste-enhancing addition to the vegetable-rich main courses," she writes. "Think of the couscous of Morocco or the thiebou dienn of Senegal. . . . Think of the millet couscous of Mali or the rice that goes under the main dish in much of Sierra Leone." Traditional African diets were rich with plant proteins such as black-eyed peas, vitamin- and mineral-filled leafy greens and high-fiber grains including rice and millet, Harris argues. Salt and sugar were eaten sparingly.

This largely plant-based diet appears to be more compatible with our genetic inheritance, according to Milton Mills, MD, assistant director of preventive medicine at the Physicians Committee for Responsible Medicine in Washington, D.C. Studies show that when African-Americans are put on plant-based diets, our rates of chronic disease start to decline. "What you see immediately is the incidence of hypertension, diabetes and obesity starts to decrease," he explains. "That argues that Blacks are genetically-adapted to a plant-based, low-fat diet." For example, a 1998 Loma Linda University study found that mildly hypertensive African-Americans who switched to potassium-rich, high-fruit diets (raisins, bananas, orange juice) for six weeks lowered their mean blood pressure significantly, more so than those who ate less fruit and vegetables.

Another reason to embrace a traditional African eating plan is that blacks have naturally higher levels of a lipoprotein known as LPa, which can increase our risk of heart disease, says Mills. Because of this tendency, we have an even greater chance of developing heart disease on a high animal-fat diet than whites eating such a diet. But on a more traditional low animal-fat diet, our risk is minimal.

Researchers all over the world are recognizing the value of the plant-based style of diet that was consumed by our West African ancestors. The Food Guide Pyramid, which was introduced by U.S. Department of Agriculture (USDA) in 1992 to replace the outdated four food groups, now weighs more heavily on grains, fruits, and vegetables and less on meat, poultry, fish, and dairy products. The healthiest diets culled from the Mediterranean all have one thing in common: a plant base. Researchers note that people who eat such diets in Mediterranean countries live longer and suffer less chronic disease than those who don't.

Choosing the Diet For *You*

But the latest study or nutrition book on the market is not as important as how a particular diet makes you feel. The key expert to consult is your own body. When Tara Harper decided to adopt a vegetarian diet three years ago, she became aware of a change. "I felt lighter," says the New York lawyer, who no longer has to go through bottles of antacids every month the way she used to. "My skin is more clear and my hair is healthier," she notes. Since giving up meat over ten years ago, Nikki DeJesus Smith of Washington, D.C., says, "I find that I am not sick with colds and allergies as often as I used to be. Now, whatever I eat fills me up and I have much more energy."

As you evaluate your diet and make adjustments to it throughout your life, pay attention to what your body is telling you.

Black Women and Weight

We need only to look around at our friends and family members to know that black women come in all beautiful shapes and sizes. However, too much weight and too little activity harm our health. In 1995, 65 percent of all black women were overweight and a disproportionate number were severely obese. Excess weight is responsible for many of our medical problems including diabetes, hypertension, and heart disease. Our healthy acceptance of varying body types may mask a potentially dangerous health problem.

If you are concerned about your weight and health, talk to your health care provider, who can help you determine whether your current weight is putting you in harm's way. If you decide that you do need to shed some pounds, resist the temptation to try fad diets that promise rapid weight loss, or diet drugs. These often lead to temporary success and long-term frustration. The only proven way to take pounds off permanently is to eat less and exercise more. "I think women have got to look at themselves and take a personal inventory," says Long Island, New York nutritionist Constance Brown-Riggs, RD. "Generally, people know what they should be doing; they don't know how. At the same time, they know what they should be doing from the outside as opposed to the inside. They have to be honest with themselves. How much excessive food are they eating? Are they skipping meals? What is their health status? That can be a motivator for change." How to do it:

• Set realistic goals. Experts agree that losing as little as five or ten pounds—and keeping them off—can provide health benefits including lowered cholesterol and blood pressure. Don't try to lose more than one pound a week.

• Consult the experts. A nutritionist can help you devise a healthy diet plan and a personal trainer can give you tips on how to exercise for weight reduction. To find a registered dietitian, ask friends and colleagues, or contact the American Dietetic Association at (800) 366-1655 or *www.eatright.org.*

• Keep a food-mood diary. For a week or a month, take note of what you eat, when, and how you are feeling. By recognizing emotional eating patterns, you can take steps to change them.

• Make one change at a time. Dramatic changes in lifestyle are often followed by relapses. Instead, make small changes over time. You might start by simply eating one more piece of fruit or a vegetable a day, says Brown-Riggs. Or add one day to your exercise regimen until it becomes a habit.

• Snack on fruits and vegetables during the day to avoid overeating at night. Always eat breakfast.

• Learn to relax. Even just ten minutes of solitude and deep breathing at the beginning and the end of your day can take the edge off stress that often leads to bingeing. Prayer will also ease anxiety.

• Be gentle with your body. The desire to be thin can alienate us from the precious temple that is our body, and fill us with feelings of inadequacy and pain. As you develop a healthier relationship to your body, treat it kindly with fragrant lotions, soothing bubble baths, and regular massages.

Self-Awareness Tool

Mood-Food Diary

For at least three days this week, take the opportunity to record your diet and mood. Note the time of day you eat, what mood you're in (happy, sad, bored, angry, silly), and what you eat and drink.

DAY 1

	Time of Day	Food/Beverage	Mood
Breakfast			
Lunch			

_____

_____

_____

Dinner

_____

_____

_____

_____

_____

Snacks

_____

_____

_____

DAY 2

	Time of Day	Food/Beverage	Mood

Breakfast

_____

_____

_____

Lunch

_____

_____

_____

_____

_____

Dinner

_____

_____

_____

_____

Snacks

_____

_____

_____

DAY 3

Time of Day	Food/Beverage	Mood

Breakfast

_____

_____

_____

_____

_____

Lunch

_____

_____

_____

_____

_____

Dinner

_____

_____

_____

_____

_____

Snacks

_____

_____

_____

At the end of three days, look over your diary. Take notes of patterns. What did you eat when you were in a good mood? Does that differ from what you ate at other times? Also take note of your overall diet: Would you say your diet was balanced during the three days? Did you skip a meal or go for several hours without eating?

If you suspect that your moods affect your dietary choices, knowing that can empower you to make different choices. Before you eat, get in the habit of bringing your mood to mind and naming it. Instead of making poor nutritional choices or skipping meals, decide what you will do when you are feeling anxious or blue. You might simply take a walk, call a friend, write in a journal, say a prayer, or breathe deeply—whatever works to calm you and put your problems in perspective. Whatever the concern, don't punish your body; learn how to nurture yourself.

If you noticed some problems in your diet—too little fruit, too much salt, or skipped meals, for example—don't let it slide. Challenge yourself to make at least one change in your diet this month. For example, you might drink two extra glasses of water per day. Then repeat the exercise. If you have questions regarding your diet, talk to your health-care provider or a nutritionist. To find a registered dietitian, ask for referrals from your provider or contact the American Dietetic Association, (800) 366-1655 or *www.eatright.org.*

Vegetarianism

Our West African ancestors were vegetarians. Despite the fact that they did not have sophisticated medical systems or pharmaceutical drugs, their largely plant-based diet was sufficient to protect them from health problems such as high blood pressure, obesity, and high cholesterol, conditions that are widespread among African-Americans today. A growing number of Americans are vegetarian, including approximately 3.5 percent of all African-Americans, according to the 2000 Vegetarian Resource Group Zogby poll. Research suggests that vegetarianism may be the best dietary choice for us. According to a study published in the *American Journal of Clinical Nutrition,*

Black Seventh-Day Adventists who ate few or no animal products had less abdominal fat, were less likely to be hypertensive, and had lower cholesterol levels than those who ate animal products daily.

Studies demonstrate that vegetarians overall have lower incidences of hypertension and colorectal cancer than nonvegetarians. They are less likely to die of diabetes complications, renal disease, and heart disease—the leading killer of African-Americans. In fact, switching to a low-fat, vegetarian eating plan, in conjunction with exercise and stress-management techniques, has been shown to halt and reverse the progression of heart disease right in its tracks.

In addition to health concerns, many vegetarians choose the lifestyle for environmental, ecological, moral, or spiritual reasons. While in graduate school DeJesus Smith was disturbed to learn about how meat was processed. "I was horrified to learn that some processing plants are allowed to use sick animals," she says. "After that, I was turned off." Environmentalists also note that the clearing of land for cattle grazing has destroyed millions of acres of tropical rainforests, and that growing feed for farm animals wastes water and land while it increases pesticide use. The overcrowding, overfeeding, and general mistreatment and abuse of chickens, hogs, and cows also trouble vegetarians. Some simply believe animals are not on this Earth for us to eat. "I'm a very spiritual person," Tara says. "Part of my comfort in not eating animals is that I think they weren't put here for me to consume." Our ancestors agreed. According to Coetzee, traditional Africans societies rarely slaughtered cattle because the animals were held in esteem and considered a means of exchange, not food.

Some nonvegetarians think that vegetarian living is too extreme and restrictive, or that the diet will be flavorless. But there are many ways to be a vegetarian, and vegetarian diets vary as much as individual vegetarians do. The most obvious difference relates to what degree each vegetarian chooses to avoid or exclude animal products from her diet. The main vegetarian types include:

Semi- or Partial or Quasi-vegetarian. Probably the most common style of vegetarian eating in the United States is a diet based mainly on vegetables, fruits, grains, legumes, seeds, nuts, dairy products, and eggs with some inclusion of chicken or fish. Some semi-vegetarians may also eat red meat on rare occasions.

Lacto-ovo-vegetarian. This type of vegetarian excludes fish, chicken, and meat entirely but continues to eat both dairy products and eggs.

Vegan or Complete Vegetarian. Vegan (pronounced "vee-gun") diets exclude all animal products, including butter. About 4 percent of all vegetarians are vegan.

Making the Transition

If you currently eat meat, but have always wanted to be a vegetarian, you can make the shift gradually. Transition tips:

- Add more vegetables and fruit to your diet. Make a list of your favorite veggies—and maybe one or two you've never tried—so you can plan to pick them up while getting groceries. Add vegetables to sandwiches and stir-fries. Stir fruit into yogurt and cereal and substitute fruit for cakes and sweets.
- Experiment with plant protein sources, including various beans, soy products, nuts, and seeds. Tara Harper enjoys baked tofu, falafel, and vegetable burgers.
- Plan meatless (no meat, chicken, or fish) meals. Start with one dinner a week, then two, and so on.
- Make vegetarian friends. You can cook vegetarian meals together or eat at vegetarian restaurants to reinforce each other's commitment.
- Buy vegetarian cookbooks such as *The Gradual Vegetarian.* Or take a class on vegetarian cooking at a local cooking school.

NATURAL WOMAN: SHANI SAXON

Like many women, 27-year-old Shani Saxon used to love eating filling comfort foods such as burgers, cakes, and cookies. But the magazine editor has also always had strong discipline. At age 13, she stopped eating red meat cold turkey in spite of the fact that she

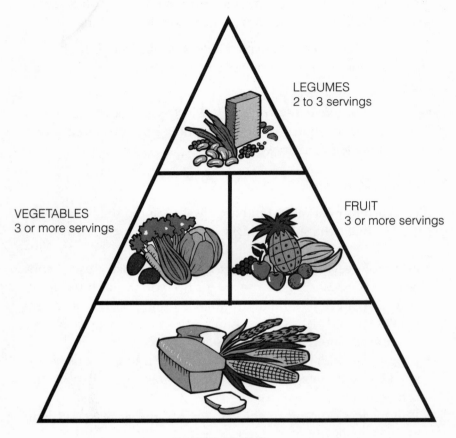

LEGUMES
2 to 3 servings

VEGETABLES
3 or more servings

FRUIT
3 or more servings

WHOLE GRAINS
5 or more servings

How to Eat Right

This vegetarian-style food pyramid illustrates the plant-based diet recommended by the Physicians Committee for Responsible Medicine. Be sure to include a good source of vitamin B_{12}.

comes from a family of carnivores. At age 21, just a few months after switching to a vegetarian diet, Shani decided to become a vegan. "I knew that if I became vegan I wouldn't cheat because it would be like going against something I believe in," she says. "I can always tell myself that a regular diet is over, but a way of life is just that. As I started reading about my new eating habits and figuring out what I could and couldn't eat, it all started to mean a lot more to me."

Over the next few months, Shani learned as much as she could about this nutritional plan that would require her to give up all foods made from animal products. She read books like The Gradual Vegetarian *and experimented with unfamiliar healthy foods like tempeh. The most difficult part of the transition was not in finding foods she liked or maintaining a high energy level, but in dealing with people who didn't understand her choice. "As soon as someone finds out I'm vegan, they usually turn into amateur nutritionists," she explains. " 'You must not get enough protein' is what I hear most often. Half the time people don't know what they're talking about."*

In the six years she's been vegan, Shani has shed ten pounds and feels great. "The best thing is being able to go to bed feeling guilt free and knowing that I did the best I could for my body that day," she says. Shani also believes that her eating style nourishes her whole self. "I realized how much we abuse our bodies and fill them with substances that not only ruin our health but cloud our minds and hurt our spirits," she notes. "[Deciding to go vegan] wasn't about staying thin anymore, it was about loving myself and respecting my body."

Commonly Asked Questions

Q. *How will I get enough protein?*
A. Look to plant sources such as beans, almonds, and sesame seeds. Nutritionists also point out that many vegetables and fruits provide sufficient protein—without all the fat of animal products.

Q. Do I have to worry about vitamin or mineral deficiencies?
A. Vegetarians who eat a variety of organic, unprocessed foods should not have to worry about deficiencies with one notable exception—vitamin B_{12}. Very little B_{12} is available in plant foods, and since a B_{12} deficiency could take years to cause symptoms, vegans and vegetarians who limit animal products should consider supplements. Because our bodies don't absorb B_{12} efficiently as we age, older vegetarians should also supplement. See the list of additional nutrients of concern to vegetarians below.

Q. Can I continue eating a vegetarian diet if I'm pregnant?
A. Yes, and during lactation as well. According to the American Dietetic Association, a carefully planned semivegetarian or vegan diet will provide enough nutrients to mother and child. To lower the risk of birth defects, however, all pregnant women are urged to supplement with folic acid. Vegan moms may want to also supplement with vitamin B_{12} because it is difficult to get enough in nonanimal foods.

Q. Can I raise my child vegetarian?
A. Yes! Well-planned vegetarian and vegan diets can meet the nutritional needs of infants and children, according to the American Dietetic Association. You can feed your vegetarian infants pureed tofu and legumes, and older kids can do quite well on diets that emphasize calcium, iron, and zinc. Vegan children may need extra vitamin B_{12} and vitamin D.

Q. Are there any risks to eating a vegetarian diet?
A. Besides potential deficiencies that can be corrected through a balanced diet and/or supplementation, vegetarian diets are generally healthier than nonvegetarian diets. In fact, there are greater risks associated with eating animal foods.

The following is a list of foods that supply iron and calcium, two nutrients that vegetarians may be lacking, according to the American Dietetic Association's website:

Iron	Calcium
Whole wheat bread, 1 slice	Chickpeas, 1 cup, cooked.
White bread (enriched), 1 slice	Great northern beans, 1 cup, cooked
Bran flakes, 1 cup	Navy beans, 1 cup, cooked
Cream of wheat, ½ cup, cooked	Pinto beans, 1 cup, cooked
Oatmeal, instant, 1 packet	Black beans 1 cup, cooked
Wheat germ, 2 tablespoons	Vegetarian baked beans,1 cup, cooked
Beet greens, ½ cup, cooked	Soybeans, 1 cup, cooked
Sea vegetables, ½ cup, cooked	Tofu, ½ cup
Swiss chard, ½ cup, cooked	Tempeh, ½ cup
Tomato juice, 1 cup	Textured vegetable protein, ½ cup
Turnip greens, ½ cup, cooked	Soy milk, 1 cup
Baked beans, vegetarian, ½ cup, cooked	Soy milk, fortified, 1 cup
Black beans, ½ cup, cooked	Soy nuts, ½ cup
Garbanzo beans, ½ cup, cooked	Almonds, 2 tablespoons
Kidney beans, ½ cup, cooked	Almond butter, 2 tablespoons
Lentils, ½ cup, cooked	Bok choy, ½ cup, cooked
Lima beans, ½ cup, cooked	Broccoli, ½ cup, cooked
Navy beans, ½ cup, cooked	Collard greens, ½ cup, cooked
Soybeans, ½ cup, cooked	Kale, ½ cup, cooked
Tempeh, ½ cup, cooked	Mustard greens, ½ cup, cooked
Tofu, ½ cup, cooked	Turnip greens, ½ cup, cooked
Soy milk, 1 cup	Dried figs, 5
Cashews, 2 tablespoons	Calcium-fortified orange juice, 1 cup
Pumpkin seeds, 2 tablespoons	Blackstrap molasses, 1 tablespoon
Tahini, 2 tablespoons	Cow's milk, 1 cup
Sunflower seeds, 2 tablespoons	Yogurt, 1 cup
Blackstrap molasses, 1 tablespoons	

Zinc	Vitamin D
Bran flakes, 1 cup	Fortified, ready-to-eat cereal, ½ cup
Wheat germ, 2 tablespoons	Fortified soy milk or nondairy milk, 1 cup
Adzuki beans, ½ cup, cooked	
Chickpeas, ½ cup, cooked	**Vitamin B$_{12}$**
Lima beans, ½ cup, cooked	Ready-to-eat cereal, ½ cup
Lentils, ½ cup,cooked	Meat substitute, 1 serving or package
Soybeans, ½ cup, cooked	Fortified soy milk or other nondairy milk, 8 ounces
Tempeh, ½ cup, cooked	Nutritional yeast, 1 tablespoon
Tofu, ½ cup, cooked	
Textured vegetable protein, ½ cup, cooked	**Linolenic acid**
Corn, ½ cup, cooked	Flax seed, 2 tablespoons
Peas, ½ cup, cooked	Walnuts, 1 ounce
Sea vegetables, ½ cup, cooked	Walnut oil, 1 tablespoon
Cow's milk, 1 cup	Canola oil, 1 tablespoon
Cheddar cheese, 1 ounce	Linseed oil, 1 tablespoon
Yogurt, 1 cup	Soybean oil, 1 tablespoon
	Soybeans, ½ cup, cooked
	Tofu, ½ cup

Additional Alternative Diets

Macrobiotic. Meaning long (macro) life (bios), macrobiotics is an ancient dietary practice based on the idea that eating the proper balance of foods will lead to a balanced and harmonious life. The foods included in this semivegetarian diet—mainly grains, beans, seeds, nuts, and root and sea vegetables, plus some fresh fish, seafood, and fruit—are all categorized by the *yin* (cooler) and *yang* (warmer) theory of opposites. Foods with too much yin or yang, including alcohol, caffeine, sugar, meat, dairy, and, processed foods, are avoided altogether. The more balanced foods should be eaten whole and in season. To preserve the balance within foods, macrobiotic practitioners use cooking methods such as steaming, flame-broiling, and pressure cooking. The lifestyle also promotes exercise and positive thinking.

Because it is a low-fat, mainly plant-based diet, macrobiotic eating has the potential for preventing and healing several health problems, including high cholesterol, high blood pressure, obesity, diabetes, arthritis, heart disease, AIDS, and cancer. Even the most carefully planned macrobiotic diet may still be deficient in key nutrients such as vitamin B_{12}, so taking supplements is often recommended, though some macrobiotic folks reject supplements as unnatural.

Blood-Type Diet

Based on the work of researchers James D'Adamo, MD, and Dr. Peter D'Adamo, the notion of creating an eating plan according to blood type has gained popularity in recent years. While studying nutrition and health in Germany during World War II, James D'Adamo developed the idea that certain foods might be more suitable for certain individuals. D'Adamo believed that blood is the source of life and that because different blood types evolved at different times, people are genetically adapted to eating what their ancestors—specifically those with the same blood type—ate. A summary of blood types and the foods D'Adamo recommends:

- Type O (50 percent of African-Americans): Eat some lean meat (chicken, turkey), fish (cod, sole), green vegetables (collards, kale); avoid whole wheat and dairy products.
- Type A (24 percent of African-Americans): Eat green vegetables, fruits (berries, figs), some grains, only lean meat and fish if any; avoid dairy products.
- Types B and AB (24 percent of African-Americans): Eat low-fat dairy; green, red, and yellow vegetables; fruit, some grains, some turkey or fish if any animal protein.

41

According to the blood-type theory, different types also have particular temperaments and needs for exercise and relaxation. Though this theory has not been proven scientifically, it does confirm the fact that most blacks—and most people—are not adapted to eating dairy products and should avoid them.

Raw Food

This vegetarian diet consists of uncooked fruits, vegetables, nuts, seeds, and sprouts; no animal products or grains. Raw food practitioners believe that food is alive and that cooking it destroys vital vitamins, minerals, fiber, and enzymes. Eating this raw vegetarian diet guarantees more nutrients and more fiber which prevents potentially harmful waste from remaining in the colon. Practitioners can juice or grate food for easier digestion. Organic produce is preferred to cut down on pesticide exposure. Because vitamin B_{12} is mainly found in animal products, raw food eaters might want to consider supplementation; talk to a nutritionist or your health care provider.

NATURAL WOMAN: NJERI JACKSON

Becoming a mother was the first incentive for Njeri Jackson, PhD, to forgo the standard American diet and experiment with healthier eating styles at the age of 19. "I became very serious about changing my diet because I wanted to make sure I had a healthy child," the 50-year-old associate professor and director of African-American studies recalls. Her second motive was political: "It was the sixties. There were a number of things going on that were encouraging people to reassess everything about American lifestyles and cultures—the Civil Rights Movement, the Women's Movement, the Environmental Movement, the Community Health Movement. At that time, there was a lot of information coming out about the dangers of a meat-based diet."

At first Njeri switched from eating the red meat at the grocery store to eating kosher meat. Over a period of three years, she gradually eliminated all animal products. By 1973, she was eating a vegan diet, a diet she maintained for a decade and a half. Then, in the late eighties, after reading books about the benefits of eating raw foods, she decided to take her quest for better health a step further. "The more I read, the clearer it became to me that the best source of nutrients was uncooked foods," she explains. "In the process of heating food, you destroy most of the vitamins and nutrients in them."

Though eating such a diet was sometimes difficult for her daughters to accept, it was natural for Njeri. "My father had been a cook in the Navy. He always used fresh fruits and vegetables at home, so I knew to eat a lot of that kind of food." Sticking to a vegan diet, eating organic, raw foods, and occasionally fasting, in addition to regular exercise, has kept Njeri in excellent health throughout her life. "Women have a high incidence of bladder and urinary infections that are closely related to diet. I haven't [had those problems] since I switched my diet. My energy levels are phenomenal."

Ayurvedic Diet

The most famous proponent of the ancient Indian Ayurvedic healing system is Deepak Chopra. This system is based on the idea that individuals have unique dietary needs determined by their constitution, or basic nature. Depending on a variety of physical and psychological characteristics, you are categorized by your dominant force or dosha—either vata (ether and air), pitta (fire and water), or kapha (water and earth). Each dosha or combination of doshas requires specific types of foods to remain balanced and healthy. Under the Ayurvedic system, foods are also categorized into six tastes (sweet, sour, salty, bitter, pungent, and astringent) and six qualities (heavy, oily, hot, light, dry, and cold).

Ayurvedic eating may not be simple. It requires you to choose specific foods to balance your dosha and to eat seasonally. But the payoff can be big: The Ayurvedic diet has the potential to treat a variety of disorders and conditions, including diabetes, arthritis, high blood pressure, coronary heart disease, just to name a few. If you are interested in learning about Ayurveda, first consult an Ayurvedic physician to determine your dosha type and prescriptive diet. (See the Resources.)

Fasting for Health

Fasting, or abstaining from food for as little as one day to as many as thirty, has long been used as a method of physical, mental, and spiritual cleansing. Your body, which sends you the message to avoid food while you have colds or the flu, knows this intuitively. Natural healers believe that first and foremost, fasting gives your body a break from the work of digestion. It is also believed that fasting helps the body detoxify, or rid itself of toxins such as pesticides and chemicals. Fasting can alleviate certain conditions (headaches, sinus problems) and potentially cure others (arthritis, diabetes, asthma, heart disease) if the practice is followed by a more permanent change in diet and lifestyle.

Fasting does not equal starvation. Though some people only drink water during a fast, others ingest fruit or vegetable juices, and still others enjoy a modified fast of just raw vegetables and fruit. Initially, your body uses stored glucose, then fat, for energy. This process can cause withdrawal symptoms—dizziness, insomnia, headache—which should subside in a day or two. Some nutritionists believe that people who have the most reactions are in the most need of a fast. But to avoid potential problems, you should only practice fasting under the care of a health provider. (People with diabetes need to watch for blood sugar reactions and check with their doctor before beginning a fast.) Pregnant women should not fast.

To assist your body during a fast, plan to gradually eliminate foods a week or two before you begin. Get plenty of rest, drink a lot of water, and consider taking a multivitamin/multimineral supplement during the fast. Some experts recommend taking specific supplements to cleanse the colon such as fiber, psyllium, and acidophilus. At the end of your fast, add foods back in as gradually as you eliminated them. A nutritionist or naturopath can help you determine what type of fast is best for you. If you enjoy the benefits of a fast, such as increased energy and mental clarity, plan to repeat it seasonally.

Diet Dilemmas

Sugar, Starch, and Diabetes

Eating large amounts of refined sugar in cakes, cookies, soda, ice cream, and other common foods can be detrimental to our health and well-being. White sugar is high in calories but devoid of nutrients. It increases our insulin levels and hampers our immune system by limiting the function of white blood cells and antibodies. Some health experts believe that glucose contributes to the growth of yeast in the body and may even also feed tumors.

White bread and rice may also be hazardous when eaten in excess. These refined grains swiftly raise our blood sugar and increase the amount of insulin in the blood. The inevitable blood sugar crash makes us feel hungry again within just a few hours. Over time, a high-refined starch diet—filled with bagels, white bread, and pasta, for example—can lead to weight gain and obesity. This combined with chronically high insulin levels can make us susceptible to developing type II diabetes.

Foods that raise our blood sugar to potentially unhealthy levels are said to have a high glycemic index or GI. These include white or whole wheat bread and pasta, white and brown rice, corn, white potatoes, carrots, common breakfast cereals, rice cakes, French fries, and soft drinks, among others. Eating an abundance of such foods over time can cause weight gain, which can lead to insulin resistance, a condition in which the body no longer responds to insulin properly. Insulin resistance has been linked to several chronic diseases, including diabetes, heart disease, and colon cancer. High glycemic foods are not inherently "bad" for you, but they must be eaten in small quantities as part of a balanced diet that includes leafy vegetables and other low glycemic foods.

The Dairy Dilemma

In spite of the fact that many of us grew up believing that milk was wholesome and good for us, most blacks—some 70 percent or more—cannot properly digest it. Though we may be able to enjoy milk as children, many of us stop making the enzyme that is needed to break down milk sugar, or lactase, in our late teens or early twenties, says Milton Mills, MD. At that point symptoms such as gas, stomach cramps, diarrhea, and bloating might occur when we drink a glass of milk or eat an ice cream cone. Many of Dr. Mills's patients who complained of conditions like irritable bowel syndrome found their symptoms disappeared once they stopped eating dairy.

The diarrhea and gas caused by lactose intolerance are good enough reasons to consider cutting dairy products such as milk, cheese, and ice cream from your diet, but there are others. Because dairy products increase mucus production in the body, they may exacerbate or contribute to allergies. Like other sources of animal protein, dairy foods are typically high in saturated fat and cholesterol, both contributors to heart disease, diabetes, and certain cancers. Cow's milk may also contain residues from the hormones and antibiotics given to cows to fatten them up and keep them infection-free; it is unclear what the health impact of those residues might be.

Black women may be advised to drink milk to keep bones strong and prevent fractures and osteoporosis. However, our bones are naturally denser than those of white and Asian women, who have higher rates of osteoporosis. And milk is not the only source of calcium. Other sources, including dark green leafy vegetables, beans, fortified soy milk, and oatmeal, offer calcium that is readily absorbed and they are superior nutritionally. Also, physical activity and avoiding smoking, caffeine, and alcohol are just as essential for calcium absorption and retention and bone health. For those of us who love the taste of certain dairy foods like cheese and ice cream, there are healthier plant-based substitutes made from soy, rice, and nuts. Lactose-reduced products are also found in stores.

Food Allergies

The foods we eat are usually a source of pleasure, but for certain folks, eating the wrong food can cause discomfort and pain. A food allergy develops when a person's immune system mistakes certain foods for enemy invaders such as viruses and germs. Eating even a tiny amount of the offending food (allergen) quickly triggers a reaction, or the release of massive amounts of chemicals intended to rid the body of the invading food. Symptoms are often severe and can be life-threatening. Unlike a food intolerance (e.g. lactose intolerance), which is triggered by eating larger amounts of food and which takes longer to cause reactions, allergic reactions occur within minutes (or even seconds) every time the offending food is eaten.

To avoid the discomfort and danger of food allergies, learn about them and be extra careful about what you eat. Take note of these food allergy facts:

Common Foods That Cause Allergies: Peanuts, tree nuts, milk, wheat, corn, eggs, fish, and shellfish.

Symptoms: Breathing problems; itchy and watery eyes; hives; sudden drop in blood pressure; nausea; vomiting; diarrhea; swelling of the lips, tongue, and throat; unconsciousness; and often anaphylaxis—a condition which can turn rapidly fatal without prompt emergency treatment.

Diagnosis: Consult your doctor or an allergist, who will prescribe skin and blood tests and/or an elimination diet to identify allergens.

Managing Allergies: Totally eliminate offending foods from the diet. Always check food labels and inquire about ingredients in menu items whenever you eat out. Inform family, coworkers, and friends of your allergy so they are aware and can be ready to help if needed, especially if you become incapacitated. People with severe reactions should always carry an epinephrine self-injector kit, which can save their life until they can get emergency care. Never ignore symptoms, and know what to do. Wear a medical alert bracelet or necklet naming your allergy.

Resources

American Dietetic Association, 216 West Jackson Boulevard, Suite 800, Chicago, IL 60606; (800) 366-1655; *www.eatright.org*

American School of Ayurvedic Sciences, Ayurvedic and Naturopathic Medical Clinic, 2115 112th Avenue, NE, Bellevue, WA 98004; *www. ayurvedicscience.com*

Ayurvedic Institute, 11311 Menaul NE, Suite A, Alburquerque, NM, 87112; *www.ayurveda.com*

Nutrition Education Association, Inc., 3647 Glen Haven Blvd., Houston, TX 77025.

Physician's Committee for Responsible Medicine, 5100 Wisconsin Avenue, NW, Suite 404, Washington DC, 20016.

Ayurvedic Cooking for Self-Healing, by Usha Lad and Vasant Lad, (Ayurvedic Press).

The Complete Book of Alternative Nutrition, by Selene Yeager, the Editors of *Prevention Magazine* Health Books, (Editor), and E. Ellis Cashmore (Editor) (Berkley).

Eat Right 4 Your Type: The Individualized Diet Solution to Staying Healthy, Living Longer and Achieving Your Ideal Weight, by Dr. Peter J. D'Adamo with Catherine Whitney (Putnam).

The Gradual Vegetarian: The Step-by Step Way to Start Eating the Right Stuff Today!, by Lisa Tracy (Dell).

Prescription for Nutritional Healing, by James F. Balch, MD, and Phyllis A. Balch CNC. (Avery).

Chapter 3

⌒

Some Added Insurance: Supplements

NATURAL WOMAN: JOYCE WHITE

Before 1997, Joyce White had never thought about taking vitamin or mineral supplements. She power-walked each morning and got a healthy dose of fruits and vegetables every day. But during a routine exam at her doctor's office, Joyce learned that both her cholesterol and blood sugar levels were elevated. In addition to urging her to continue her good eating-and-exercise habits, Joyce's health care provider suggested she take a few supplements as well, including vitamin E and folic acid to strengthen the heart and chromium picolinate to lower the risk of diabetes. In a matter of months, Joyce's new health regimen produced positive results: Her blood sugar returned to normal and her cholesterol count dropped several points.

More recently, Joyce has added new pills as part of her daily bread. Her supplement cocktail now includes a multivitamin containing the heart-friendly vitamin E and folic acid and gugulipids, a supplement derived from the Indian gum tree that is purported to help lower cholesterol naturally. She also occasionally consumes brewer's yeast in juice to get her B vitamins. For other nutrients, Joyce makes sure to eat a lot of green vegetables, fresh fruit, and fish. To keep abreast of the potential benefits and risks of taking various supplements, she reads health magazines and articles in newspapers. Besides her concern about her cholesterol creeping up, the 55-year-old feels fit and in control of her health.

Folic acid. Flaxseed oil. Vitamin E. You've probably heard about these nutrients or included one in your daily supplement regimen. While our mothers and grandmothers may have used vitamin C to curb a cold, the range of supplements commonly used today is ever-increasing. These days, many people take supplements daily or at least on occasion to prevent or combat a particular ailment or to simply improve their health. The more medical science learns about the therapeutic value of vitamins, minerals, and other nutrients, the more supplements are being recognized as powerful natural healing tools.

Supplementing Our Health

What we know as dietary or nutritional supplements include vitamins, minerals, enzymes, amino acids, antioxidants, phytochemicals, and even hormones. (Herbs are also sold as "supplements." We'll explore them in Chapter 4.) Among the most popular supplements, and the ones that have been researched most, are vitamins and minerals. Once used mainly for the prevention of severe nutritional deficiencies, supplements are being researched for their potential to help prevent and treat numerous health problems, from premenstrual syndrome and birth defects to heart disease and cancer.

Though experts in nutrition agree that food is a far superior source of the nutrients our bodies need to function at their best, they also say supplements can be helpful for several reasons. While there's evidence that our early ancestors received more than enough of the nutrients they needed to survive through the food they gathered and hunted, we are not as fortunate. The quality of the food many of us eat today is nutritionally inferior for many reasons. Chemically fertilized soil does not contain as many nutrients as soil fertilized naturally, says Milton Mills, a Washington D.C.-based internist specializing in nutrition. Plants grown in this soil don't receive the abundance and variety of nutrients they would from soil fertilized organically with manure or decaying leaves. "If you've ever tasted an organic potato versus a conventional one, it's immediately apparent that the organic version has more intense flavor," Mills explains. Commercial farms also limit their produce to strains that are chosen for high yield and appearance, further diminishing their nutrient potential.

The quality of the food in our grocery stores is further threatened by developments such as genetic engineering and irradiation, says Jewel Pookrum, MD, PhD, an Atlanta-based gynecologist who specializes in integrative medicine. Today, an innocent-looking strawberry in your produce aisle may have been genetically engineered to resist frost. A bright yellow banana from Honduras may have been artificially ripened in a laboratory without soil or sunlight. Other foods may be irradiated by the same agent used in cancer therapy. Truth be told, these modern techniques have unknown effects on our foods and unknown effects on our bodies. The shipping, storage, and processing of foods also rob them of their natural vitamin and mineral content. Buying and eating such foods, Pookrum contends, creates, at the very least, the potential for unknown nutritional deficiencies.

Even if we all switched to shopping in organic supermarkets today, few of us can say we eat a well-balanced diet every single day, or even on most days. Many busy women don't make time for a full breakfast, much less a day's worth of complete meals that contain the range of vitamins and minerals our bodies need. Chopping, slicing, and cooking foods diminish their nutritional value further. "Very few people get well-prepared, well-balanced meals," says Mills. Today many experts agree that the amount of nutrients recommended for optimal health would be nearly impossible to get through diet alone.

Add to these arguments the fact that our bodies are drained of vitamins and minerals whenever we get sick, take pharmaceutical drugs, absorb environmental pollutants, or face undue stress. Each of these factors keeps our bodies working overtime, drawing on precious vitamin and minerals stores, just to stay afloat. Given that a high percentage of black women live in polluted urban areas with limited access to fresh foods, labor for long hours in stressful, unhealthy workplaces, and suffer disproportionately from health problems, we may be prime candidates for supplementation.

NATURAL WOMAN: ALLISON ABNER

Television writer Allison Abner first took vitamin and flouride supplements as a child growing up in California. Later, as an adult, she started taking supplements again. "After college, I lost a lot of weight," she explains. "I was working really hard and I was pretty stressed out." She went to see an MD who specialized in nutrition. He gave her a blood test and found that Allison, who wasn't eating enough, was deficient in several nutrients. He started her on a course of vitamins which she stayed on for a year.

Over the next few years, Allison continued to learn more about nutrition and how she could get the nutrients her body needed through food and supplements. When she married and got pregnant, she took prenatal vitamins with folic acid to prevent birth defects. But it wasn't until her father was diagnosed with cancer in 1996 that Allison developed a more permanent supplement regimen based on the one prescribed to her father. The regimen includes a multivitamin, vitamins C and E, gingko biloba, and green tea. She's also added calcium to protect her bones and allay PMS symptoms after reading about the mineral's benefits in news reports. "PMS has really affected my mood," she says. "I have a very short cycle; I get my period every 21 days. So that means I'm PMSing half the time." Allison has also tried St. John's wort and kava kava to help manage her mood swings. How have the supplements made a difference? "I have much more energy and more even moods. I don't have menstrual cramping. My cravings for sweets are minimized."

Though we rarely hear of people developing illnesses such as rickets or scurvy that result from severe nutritional deficiencies, mild deficiencies are common. According to U.S. Department of Agriculture data, 40 percent of Americans typically get only 60 percent of the recommended daily allowance (RDA) of selected nutrients. The signs of certain deficiencies are subtle or slow to develop. We may simply feel fatigued from not getting enough iron, for example. Chronic deficiencies can result in problems ranging from anemia to depression.

But perhaps more important than how we might be harmed by a lack of vitamins and minerals is how we might be helped by a healthy supply of them. Although the knowledge we have about what specific nutrients do and how much is needed to incur health benefits is incomplete, we do know that supplements—combined with a healthy diet and exercise plan—can substantially improve our health and help stop the chain of negative events that can lead to disease. But before we start popping the latest pill mentioned in newspaper headlines or advertised at our health-food store, we should learn as much as we can about how to use supplements wisely.

How Much Is Enough? Or Too Much?

For decades, the Department of Agriculture based its recommended daily allowances, or RDAs, on what experts believed the average person needed to prevent severe nutritional deficiencies and related diseases such as rickets or beriberi. For the past several years, researchers at the National Academy of Sciences have been updating the recommendations—now called dietary reference intakes (DRIs)—to reflect what they believe individuals need to reduce the risk of the biggest threats to our health today—chronic conditions such as heart disease, cancer, and osteoporosis. These DRIs estimate average nutritional needs for men, women, and people in different age groups. They also pinpoint the levels at which specific supplements can cause harm. Because government figures tend to be conservative, nutritionist Shari Lieberman, PhD (see Resources) prefer to think in terms of optimal daily intakes, or ODIs. These describe the amounts of nutrients we need not just to survive but to thrive and combat particular health problems.

However, RDAs, DRIs, and ODIs do not take into account the particular nutritional needs of African-Americans. For example: "It's known that the African woman has ten times the bone density of Caucasian women," says Pookrum, "therefore, she needs far *more* minerals, far more calcium from plant sources." Consequently, general recommendations for calcium intake may be inadequate for sisters.

Also, depending on your age, health status, lifestyle, and family health history, you might need more of a particular nutrient or set of nutrients. For example, as you age, your body loses the ability to absorb certain nutrients such as vitamin B_{12}. Some people have metabolic disorders that prevent them from absorbing or retaining specific nutrients in adequate amounts. Having a serious illness or a family tendency toward an illness may also increase your need for supplementation. These are all good reasons to talk to a health care provider who is knowledgeable about nutrition and/or a nutritionist about your diet and supplement regimen.

Getting too much of a vitamin, mineral, or other micronutrient is a concern, but overdosing on supplements is rare. To experience adverse effects from too much of a good thing, you would have to take megadoses of a supplement over a long period of time. A greater concern is imbalance. Vitamins and minerals work synergistically. Vitamin E enhances the effects of vitamin C, for example, and vitamin D facilitates calcium absorption. However, because nutrients compete in the body for absorption, too much of one can interfere with the assimilation of another, triggering a deficiency. For example, taking too much vitamin B_6 can trigger a vitamin B_2 deficiency, since they are both absorbed by the same receptor in the intestines. And calcium interferes with the absorption of magnesium, which is also important for bone health. That's why you should avoid taking single vitamins and minerals without also taking a multivitamin or multimineral supplement for balance.

Supplement Strategies

As you investigate and incorporate supplements into your natural health plan, remember to:

- Change your diet *first*. Eat at least three meals a day, including five to nine servings of fresh vegetables and two to four servings of fruits, plus whole grains and legumes. A supplement cannot make up for a poor diet!
- Talk to your health care provider about it. Get a checkup to determine your health status and risks based on lifestyle habits and family history. Discuss any medications you are currently taking.
- Begin with a multivitamin/mineral supplement.
- Seek information about supplements. Experts are learning more about vitamins and minerals every day. Read books (see the Resources) and health magazines to keep up with the latest research.
- Be careful with dosages. Take supplements as directed on labeling. Learn about the potential toxic levels of specific vitamins and minerals.

Self-Awareness Tool

What's in Your Natural Health Cabinet?

Before you continue with or consider taking supplements, take an inventory of all the pills, potions, powders, and medications you are using on a regular basis or occasionally. This will not only help you rid your cabinet of expired products—and provide you with a list of substances that may or may not interact with each other (see "Nutrient/Drug Interactions")—but give you current information to share with your health care provider or a nutritionist. My cabinet included vitamin C, echinacea, iron, and menthol-eucalyptus lozenges, among other items. Make your list below:

_____

_____

_____

_____

_____

_____

_____

Nutrient/Drug Interactions

Common over-the-counter and prescription drugs can interfere with the absorption of vitamins and minerals. Use the following table to determine when you might need supplementation, but talk to your health care provider first.

Drug Type	Examples	Affected Vitamin or Mineral
Antacid	Aluminum hydroxide, sodium bicarbonate	Calcium, copper, folate
Antiinflammatory	Aspirin	Folate, iron, vitamin C
Antihypertensive	Hydralazine	Vitamin B_6
Diuretics		Vitamin B_2, magnesium, potassium
Hypocholesterolemia	Cholestyramine	Folate, vitamin A, vitamin B_{12}, Vitamin K
Oral contraceptives		Vitamin B_6

Vitamins and Minerals

Vitamins, minerals, and other micronutrients are essential to the proper functioning of every process of the body. These nutrients act as coenzymes, meaning they work with the body's enzymes to help it execute all of our bodily functions. Without sufficient vitamins and minerals, critical chemical reactions cannot occur. Energy cannot be released from food, nerve impulses cannot be transmitted, blood and bone cannot be formed. The vitamins and minerals we consume literally become part of us—our cells, blood, muscles, and bone—until they are utilized and needed again. Without them, the body falls out of balance, leading to diminished well-being and increased illness.

Compared to the major nutrients—carbohydrates, proteins, fats, and water—these micronutrients are needed in only small amounts. But the functions they perform, from transporting oxygen to transmitting messages across nerves, are vital to our physical *and* emotional well-being.

Some vitamins remain in our bodies for a short period of time and must be replaced daily. These are known as water-soluble vitamins and include vitamin C. Other vitamins are stored in fatty tissue for longer periods. These fat-soluble vitamins include vitamins A, D, E, and K. Minerals your body needs in large quantities are called bulk minerals or macrominerals; they include calcium, potassium, and phosphorus. Trace minerals or microminerals, needed in much smaller amounts, include copper, iron, and zinc.

Though each vitamin and mineral has a particular function or functions, as explained below, it's important to remember that these nutrients work together, enhancing each other's effects. The following nutrient intake recommendations are for women, and when indicated, for pregnant (*) or postmenopausal (**) women. ODIs are given in brackets.

Nutrient	Essential for	RDA or DRI vs. ODI (in brackets)	Food Source(s)
Vitamins			
Vitamin A and beta-carotene	Eye and skin health, immune system functions, cancer, prevention	5,000 IU [5,000–50,000 IU]	Fish liver oils, animal livers, green vegetables
Vitamin B₁ (thiamine)	Carbohydrate metabolism (energy), brain function, growth, disease prevention	1.5 mg (1.7 mg*) [25–300 mg]	Whole grains, egg yolk, legumes, fish
Vitamin B₂ (riboflavin)	Red blood cell function, eye health, carbohydrate metabolism (energy)	1.7 mg (2 mg*) [25–300 mg]	Spinach, fish, yogurt, cheese, eggs, meat
Vitamin B₃ (niacin, niacinamide, nicotonic acid)	Skin health, nervous system function, fat metabolism, digestion	20 mg [25–300mg]	Broccoli, whole wheat, cheese, fish, meat
Vitamin B₅ (pantothenic acid)	Tolerance of physical and emotional stress, immune function, fat metabolism	10 mg [25–500 mg]	Vegetables, saltwater fish, eggs, beans
Vitamin B₆ (pyrodoxine)	Nervous system function, red blood cell formation, immune function, cell growth	2 mg [25–300 mg]	Spinach, peas, walnuts, fish, eggs
Vitamin B₁₂ (cyanocobalamin)	Red blood cell formation, nervous system function (memory), cell longevity	6 mcg (8 mg*) [25–500 mcg]	Kidney, liver, herring, clams, eggs, milk

Nutrient	Essential for	RDA or DRI vs. ODI (in brackets)	Food Source(s)
Biotin	Cell growth, metabolism, healthy hair, skin, nerve tissue, and bone marrow	300 mcg [300 mcg]	Brewer's yeast soy beans, saltwater fish, meat
Choline	Nerve function, fat and cholesterol metabolism	No RDA/DRI [25–500 mg]	Legumes, whole grain cereals, eggs
Folic acid	Healthy cell division and replication, immunity, energy, fetal development	400 mcg [800 mcg*] [400–1,200 mcg]	Green leafy vegetables, wheat, liver
Inositol	Fat and cholesterol metabolism, hair growth	No RDA/DRI [25–500 mg]	Fruits, vegetables, whole grains, milk
PABA (para-aminobenzoic acid)	Folic acid formation, protein metabolism, sunburn protection (topically)	No RDA/DRI [25–500 mg]	Whole grains, liver, kidney molasses
Vitamin C (ascorbic acid)	Immune function, tissue growth and repair, stress tolerance, cancer prevention, cholesterol control	60 mg [500–5,000 mg]	Berries, citrus fruits, green vegetables
Vitamin D	Bone and teeth development, calcium absorption, immune function	400 IU 400–800 IU	Fish liver oils, fatty saltwater fish, fortified dairy products
Vitamin E	Circulation, tissue repair, blood clotting, protection of cells and fat-soluble vitamins from oxidation	30 IU [400–1,200 IU]	Natural vegetable oils, dark leafy veggies, legumes, nuts

Nutrient	Essential for	RDA or DRI vs. ODI (in brackets)	Food Source(s)
Vitamin K	Blood clotting, bone formation and repair, liver function	80 mcg [80 mcg]	Broccoli, cabbage, spinach, liver

Minerals

Nutrient	Essential for	RDA or DRI vs. ODI (in brackets)	Food Source(s)
Boron	Bone health, immune function	No RDA/DRI [3–6 mg**] No ODI	Vegetables, fruits, nuts
Calcium	Bone and tooth health, blood clotting, nerve function, muscle health	1,000 mg (1,300 mg*–1,500 mg**) [1,000–1,500 mg]	Green leafy vegetables, salmon, milk
Chromium	Glucose metabolism and blood sugar stability, cholesterol control	120 mcg [200–600 mcg]	Brewer's yeast, whole grains, cheese
Copper	Hemoglobin production, energy, nerve function, healthy bone, skin, hair	2 mg [0.5–2 mg]	Raisins, legumes, nuts, seafood, liver
Iodine	Thyroid function, physical/mental development, metabolism	150 mcg [150–300 mcg]	Kelp, seafood, saltwater fish, iodized salt
Iron	Hemoglobin production, oxidation of cells, immune function, energy	18 mg [15–30 mg]	Liver, fish, leafy veggies, whole grains
Magnesium	Bone growth, muscle function, mental health, nerve function, energy	400 mg (450 mg*) [500–750 mg]	Soybeans, nuts, seeds, seafood dairy, meat

Nutrient	Essential for	RDA or DRI vs. ODI (in brackets)	Food Source(s)
Manganese	Metabolism, bone growth, nerve function, blood sugar balance, immune function	2 mg [15–30 mg]	Seaweed, avocado, nuts, whole grains
Phosphorus	Bone and tooth strength, energy, RNA/DNA, cell function, pH balance	1,000 mg (1,300 mg*) [200–400 mg]	Whole grains, nuts, fish, dairy, meat
Potassium	Blood pressure stability, water balance, cell function, nerve transmission	No RDA/DRI [99–300 mg]	Fruit, veggie, whole grains, fish, dairy
Selenium	Immune function, cancer prevention, heart and liver function, tissue elasticity	70 mcg [50–400 mcg]	Whole grains, Brazil nuts, tuna, liver
Zinc	RNA/DNA synthesis, growth, reproduction, taste and smell, immune function	15 mg [22.5–50 mg]	Whole grains, legumes, fish, poultry, meat

(Sources: National Academy of Sciences and *The Real Vitamin and Mineral Book* by Shari Lieberman, PhD.)

NATURAL WOMAN: WENDY WEBB

Wendy Webb took multivitamins as a teen who played sports but she didn't get serious about taking supplements until she became a flight attendant. "The time zones were killing me!" says the 32-year-old. When pharmaceutical remedies left her feeling like a zombie, Wendy first tried melatonin. That led to her experimenting with other supplements. Today, she takes a combination of pills, including a women's multi which contains 37 nutrients, vitamin C, chromium picolinate ("I have cousins that had diabetes"), vitamin E, beta-carotene, and a cocktail of herbs.

"I feel great!" she says. "I like the fact that I don't have to feel overmedicated. I am always extremely busy and the energy difference is noticeable if I don't take my vitamins."

Supplement Shopping and Storage

You've walked into a health food or drug store to find rows and rows of supplement products. How do you know which brand or formula is best for the natural health benefit you seek? Some rules of thumb:

- Look for "natural" supplements. Natural supplements are derived from food; synthetic supplements are produced in laboratories. However, many "natural" supplements contain synthetic ingredients. The benefit of choosing natural formulas is to avoid the preservatives, artificial coloring, coal tars, starches, and sugars found in many synthetic brands.
- Know the lingo. Many mineral supplements will be labeled "chelated," which means the mineral is coated with a protein to enhance absorption. While absorption may be improved, chelated supplements cost more, so you'll have to decide if it's worth the investment. "Time-released" supplements are designed to dissolve slowly in the body in order to increase absorption; however, no research has proven this benefit. "Therapeutic" supplements contain doses several times greater than the daily value to maximize health benefits. But more is not always better for each individual, so be sure to stay within the range of optimum daily intake (see the table on pages 58-61) unless otherwise directed by a qualified health practitioner.
- Opt for capsules over tablets, which are inferior in

quality because they contain fillers and have been subjected to heat during the compression of the tablet.

- Shop for supplements that go down easy. Some supplements can cause nausea or constipation. Look for products that contain ingredients to counter these effects. For example, iron supplements labeled "elemental."

- Check for an expiration date. Vitamins and mineral supplements lose potency over time. To avoid taking supplements with diminished effectiveness or ones that have spoiled, buy products with expiration dates.

- Store supplements safely. Heat, cold, and moisture may affect supplements. Safer storage spots include dry, cool places or an opaque carrying container that closes tightly. Refrigeration is acceptable; in fact, all oils should be refrigerated once they're opened.

Additional Selected Supplements

Amino Acids

Known as the "building blocks" of protein, amino acids are either consumed through the diet (essential amino acids) or produced by the body (nonessential amino acids). Amino acids are linked in groups to form proteins that perform various bodily functions. Without certain amino acids, vitamins and minerals cannot be utilized effectively and the brain cannot send and receive messages. Among the twenty-eight commonly known amino acids, a few stand out in their proven ability to help the body heal when taken in supplement form. L-carnitine has been shown to boost physical stamina, increase levels of HDL (or "good") cholesterol, and protect the heart. Best known for suppressing herpes outbreaks, L-lysine can also increase calcium absorption—and bone health—in women. N-acetyl-cysteine (NAC) is an antioxidant that is beneficial in the treatment of HIV/AIDS and asthma, as well as in the prevention of age-related eye disorders and heart disease. RDIs for many amino acids have not been established, so take them only under the guidance of a licensed health care provider.

Brewer's Yeast

A basic ingredient in beer, brewer's yeast is a good source of several vitamins and minerals. Research has indicated that when taken as a supplement, brewer's yeast can not only help stabilize the blood sugar of diabetics, but also lower the risk of diabetes in folks with strong family histories of the disease. Also known as nutritional yeast, it may boost energy levels and the immune system. The daily value is 120 micrograms. It can be taken in juice or water. Avoid if you have candidiasis.

Coenzyme Q10

Present throughout the body, this vitamin-like antioxidant is believed to have multiple benefits in addition to its role in energy production. In studies, CoQ10 supplementation has been effective in the treatment of several heart-related problems, including angina, congestive heart failure, and arrhythmia. It may also help reduce risk factors for heart disease such as high blood pressure and high cholesterol. CoQ10 may also help improve symptoms in people with chronic fatigue syndrome, muscular dystrophy, and even age-related disorders. Experts have not established a daily intake recommendation for CoQ10 but good food sources include sardines, whole grains, and organ meats such as hearts.

DHEA

Secreted by the adrenal glands, this hormone is converted by the body into male and female hormones. It has many functions including immune system support, but it is best known for its antiaging potential. DHEA and related hormones decline in the body after age 25. In one study, supplementation improved the sense of well-being among 84 percent of the women who participated. It can increase muscle strength, joint comfort, and sound sleep in seniors. DHEA may also be beneficial for women with lupus. DHEA can cause unpleasant side effects including acne, hair growth, and voice changes so have your health-care provider test your hormone levels to make sure you actually are deficient. It is most effective in the dosage required and in people age 60 or older.

Essential Fatty Acids

Experts believe Greenland Eskimos have low rates of heart disease because they consume an abundance of these healthy fats in fish. Essential fatty acids (EFAs) are divided into two groups: omega-3 and omega-6 fatty acids. They protect the heart by thinning the blood naturally. In fact, fish oil supplements may be as good for heart attack prevention as aspirin, but without side effects. EFAs are also beneficial for inflammatory conditions such as asthma, rheumatoid arthritis, and lupus. One of the omega-6 fatty acids, evening primrose oil, has been proven effective for treating PMS. EFAs may also help reduce symptoms of fibrocystic breasts and painful periods. Oils from fish and seafood such as salmon, mackerel, and shrimp are the best sources of omega-3; vegetable oils supply omega-6. There is no specific recommendation for EFAs; talk to a health care provider before taking supplements.

Fiber

We've all heard that fiber is good for us for many reasons. This undigested nutrient fights disease naturally by speeding up waste removal. Scientific evidence shows that fiber rushes cholesterol out of the body, lowering the risk of heart disease. It also prevents the sharp rises in blood sugar that can lead to diabetes. By increasing stool, it prevents toxin-containing waste from staying in the colon long enough to be absorbed and perhaps trigger diseases such as colon cancer. Fiber-rich foods include whole grain cereals and breads, brown rice, beans, vegetables, and fruit. You can get the 20 to 35 daily grams of fiber recommended by the ADA by eating bran cereal in the morning, chickpeas or kidneys beans in a salad at lunch, and some broccoli or spinach with dinner. Fiber supplements can interfere with medication or other supplements, so take separately.

Lactobacillus acidophilus

Known as one of the "friendly" bacteria, lactobacillus acidophilus is commonly used by women to prevent yeast infections but it has other uses. *L. acidophilus* supplements help restore the healthy balance of bacteria in the colon as well, preventing bloating, constipation, and toxicity in the intestines that could lead to gastrointestinal cancer. If you have frequent yeast infections or take antibiotics or hormone therapy, acidophilus supplements are useful. An added benefit for blacks: Acidophilus helps our bodies digest the lactose in milk and other dairy products. A source of *L. acidophilus* is yogurt with live cultures. If you don't like yogurt or have trouble with recurrent yeast infections, look for supplements or powder in your health food store.

Melatonin

Best known as a sleep aid for insomniacs and frequent fliers, the hormone melatonin is naturally produced in the body but declines with age. Because it is secreted by the pineal gland in response to darkness and light, melatonin can help reset an off-kilter body clock and improve sleep without causing drowsiness. As an antioxidant and immune system stimulant, it also can help prevent the free radical damage that contributes to health problems such as heart disease, cataracts, and other disorders that develop with age. In studies, it has been shown to enhance the effects of anticancer drugs. Because it is a hormone that influences other hormones, melatonin may relieve symptoms of PMS and menopause, but too much of the supplement can decrease fertility. It is safest to use melatonin to address specific problems and not as a daily supplement. Food sources include rice, barley, and corn. There is no RDI, but the ODI is 1–8 mg.

Phytochemicals

If an apple a day keeps the doctor away, it may be because apples contain phytochemicals. Also known as phytomins and phytonutrients, phytochemicals are substances that give plant foods their natural color, flavor, and resistance to disease. Researchers have discovered thousands of phytochemicals in a variety of plant foods. Studies indicate a lowered risk of disease in people who eat phytochemical-rich diets. These substances work in a variety of ways. For example, flavonoids prevent the oxidation of cholesterol that leads to hardened arteries. One particular flavonoid, quercetin, is the phytochemical found in red wine that keeps blood platelets from sticking and forming clots; it may also be useful for fighting infections, inflammation, and allergies. Another flavonoid, genistein, works as a phytoestrogen, protecting the body from other forms of estrogen that trigger PMS, fibrocystic breast disease, endometriosis, menopausal symptoms, and breast cancer. Carotenoids, including beta carotene, are another type of phytochemical that prevents cell damage. Studies show that people who consume large amounts of foods containing the cartenoid lycopene have lower rates of several forms of cancer. Additional phytochemicals include indoles, isoflavones, linolenic acid, and sulforaphane. The best sources of phytochemicals are red, yellow, green, and orange fruits and vegetables, nuts, legumes, grains, onions, and wine. The ODI is 250–1,000 mg.

Supplement Cures for Conditions That Affect Us

A particular mineral or vitamin may be helpful in fortifying the body and helping to prevent—along with a healthy diet and exercise regimen—a given condition that commonly ails us. For convenience, a high-potency multivitamin/mineral may contain adequate amounts of some of the recommended nutrients. If you have a chronic medical condition, *always consult your health care provider before taking supplements.*

Ailment	Supplement	Daily Dosage
High blood pressure	Vitamin C	1 g
	Vitamin E	400 IU
	Magnesium with calcium	500 mg
		250 mg
Diabetes	Vitamin C	250 mg
	Magnesium	300 mg
	Zinc	5 mg
Asthma	B-complex	50 mg
	Magnesium with calcium	1,500 mg
		750 mg
Stress	Magnesium	200–400 mg
	B-complex	50–100 mg

Antioxidants: Nutrition All-Stars

You've probably heard about the wonders of antioxidant vitamins, minerals, and enzymes. To understand the role of antioxidants, you must first understand free radicals and the havoc they wreak in the body. Free radicals are unstable atoms that are released in the body as a result of exposure to toxic chemicals, radiation, and sunlight as well as from the metabolism of food for energy. These atoms pair with other atoms or molecules and damage or oxidize cells. In abundance, these free radicals can cause "oxidative stress," a level of cell damage that experts believe triggers several health problems including arthritis, atherosclerosis (hardened arteries), and cancer as well as aging.

To combat free radical activity, the body unleashes free radical scavengers, including certain enzymes, that block cell damage or repair it. In addition to the body's own defenses, antioxidant nutrients such as vitamins C and E keep free radical damage in check. Studies have shown that antioxidant supplements can help reduce free radicals and lower the risk of many degenerative diseases. Antioxidant vitamins and minerals include

Coenzyme Q10
Selenium
Vitamin A
Beta-carotene
Vitamin C
Vitamin E
Zinc

Resources

Africanamericanhealth.com, 220 East 26th St., Suite. 1B, New York, NY 10010; (888) 313-3103; *www.africanamericanhealth.com*

American Dietetic Association, 216 West Jackson Boulevard, Suite 800, Chicago, IL 60606; (800) 366-1655; *www.eatright.org*

Nutrition Education Association, Inc. 3647 Glen Haven, Houston, TX 77025.

Physicians' Committee for Responsible Medicine, 5100 Wisconsin Avenue, NW, Suite 404, Washington, DC 20016.

The Complete Book of Alternative Nutrition: Powerful New Ways to Use Food Supplements, Herbs and Special Diets to Prevent and Cure Disease, by the Editors of Prevention Magazine Health Books (Berkeley).

Prescription for Nutritional Healing: A Practical A-Z Reference to Drug-Free Remedies Using Vitamins, Minerals, Herbs and Food Supplements, by James F. Balch MD, and Phyllis A. Balch (Avery).

The Real Vitamin & Mineral Book, by Shari Lieberman, PhD, and Nancy Bruning (Avery).

Vitamins and Minerals from A to Z with Ethno-conciousness, by Jewel Pookrum, MD, PhD (A + B Books).

Chapter 4

~

Back to Our Roots: Healing with Herbs

NATURAL WOMAN: TREVY McDONALD

Trevy McDonald first experimented with herbal healing upon the suggestion of her health-conscious father. "He's always been into herbs, the medicinal value of plants," she says. "He would always go to the health-food store to find something." When Trevy was in need of more energy while in graduate school, he recommended ginseng. It worked, giving her the boost she needed one day to move furniture and several boxes, make a pot of shrimp Creole, and bake a cake—all with stamina to spare for her studies. Years later, Trevy decided to try herbs again to cope with her sinus problems. "I don't like taking medicine," explains the 30-year-old college professor, who lives in Chicago. "The doctor gave me a prescription decongestant and it made me nauseous. So I started blending herbal teas." Brewing and drinking cherry and peppermint tea, with eucalyptus honey for taste, knocks the sinus pressure out—without side effects.

Trevy added more natural remedies to her regimen when she learned she had fibroid tumors in 1998. To relieve her fibroid symp-

71

toms, including heavy bleeding, she started taking essiac tea, also known as floressence, and the supplement quercetin. Coincidentally, the quercetin also helps with her sinus symptoms.

As Trevy continued to learn about herbs and health by consulting alternative health practitioners, books and sources on the Internet, she also decided to eliminate meat, pork, dairy, caffeine and sugar from her diet. "I saw a difference in doing that. I don't get PMS. I lost twenty-five pounds in six weeks." She used to have sinus problems daily; now the 30-year-old professor and writer only takes her herbal medicine as needed.

Herbs for Healing

Following the tradition of our mothers and their mothers before them, many black women turn to herbs at the first sign of a cold, infection, or other ailment. The use of the clear gel inside the aloe vera plant to treat burns, or garlic to prevent infections, is not uncommon in black households, though not as common as it used to be. Black women in America relied on plant medicines for healing long before it was fashionable, but many of us are just discovering this natural healing art.

Derived from the leaves, stems, bark, roots, and flowers of plants, herbs are remarkable natural healing tools. Herbal remedies simply help the body help itself. When we apply herbal formulas to the skin in oils or poultices, or ingest them in teas or capsules, we allow compounds in herbs to work with our body chemistry in the process of healing. Unlike many pharmaceutical drugs, herbal medicines stimulate the body's natural healing capacity rather than suppressing symptoms or weakening the mind-body system. Used properly, herbs can affect mild and serious illness without troublesome side effects.

Natural Healing Is Our Heritage

For our West African ancestors, the plants growing around them served many functions—as condiments, medicines, poisons, and even agents of magic. The tropical environment produced a particularly diverse assortment of plant species, and quite naturally, traditional African societies experimented with these botanical medicines. "In the continent of Africa, the application of herbs for internal and external uses has always been a major factor in the practice of medicine," wrote Edward S. Ayensu, the Ghanaian author of *Medicinal Plants of West Africa*. "The treatment of wounds with concoctions prepared from leaves, bark and roots is a daily occurrence in an African community." The traditional use of many such herbs for specific conditions has also held up under scientific scrutiny when researchers at the Centre for Scientific Research into Plant Medicine in Ghana have tested them in clinical trials.

Some of the herbs our ancestors used made it to these shores. "Our ancestors did not come here empty-handed," says A. Kweku Andoh, PhD, ethnobotanist and founder of All African Healing Arts Society in Atlanta. "They came here in most cases with some of their own herbs." Those herbs, according to Dr. Andoh, include pidgeon pea, which was used to treat sickle-cell anemia and wild yam (*dioscorea*), an herb used for, among other things, female problems such as menstrual cramps. Those plants were particularly beneficial to Africans, says Andoh, because they were already in their systems, in their bloodstreams. What they lacked in terms of their own native herbs, they replaced with similar plants found in the New World and introduced to them by Native Americans. "When they came here, some of the elders were able to correlate the look and fragrance of certain herbs and determine how those herbs could be used to treat certain diseases," Andoh explains.

Herbal medicine is the staple of treatment in many developed and developing countries. Chinese, Indian, and Native American healers have centuries-old traditions of using plant remedies. Indeed, some 80 percent of the world's population rely on the preventive and curative powers of herbs. One quarter of all pharmaceutical drugs in the United States are derived from plants. Today herbs form an integral part of the healing practices of naturopaths, acupuncturists, and other natural healers.

Herbal Basics

You may know that ginseng gives us a boost, while valerian helps us sleep. But how, exactly, do herbs work? To understand this mystery, we must first understand that our ancestors evolved consuming plants. "First of all herbs are food," says Andoh. "They are a constituent that the body can absorb and use." Each plant contains hundreds and maybe thousands of compounds, including vitamins, minerals, and other substances, that the body can recognize and use to heal. The herb licorice is said to contain at least six hundred compounds. Knowing this begins to explain why it may be used for everything from coughs to hot flashes to vaginal infections. In many cases, scientists have discovered the active principle or principles of a particular herb. But in many other cases, much more research is needed to fully understand, how, for example, echinacea boosts the immune system.

Used singularly or in combination, herbs have multiple effects on the body. Because, according to Andoh, each plant is a "chemical factory," one herb may have multiple healing properties. Goldenseal has both antibiotic and antiseptic properties. Kava kava has sedative and aphrodisiac properties. Ginger is both a carminitive (relieves gas) and a stimulant. Practitioners also use herbs to purify the blood of excess acids and toxins, tone the organs and organ systems, and balance body fluids (diuresis), among others therapeutic purposes.

Using Herbs

If you have never used herbs before, talk to a well-trained practitioner—either a licensed herbalist, naturopathic physician, acupuncturist, chiropractor, or other experienced holistic healer. You can also talk to knowledgeable clerks in natural food stores and read some of the many books on herbs on the market to increase your own knowledge. However, if an herb or herbal formula you try does not bring about a desired effect within a few days or weeks, or causes unwanted effects, seek the guidance of a practitioner.

If you choose to use herbs on your own, you can find the herbs you need in natural health food stores, and today, many national drug-stores offer rows of herbal products. For convenience, you can buy commercially prepared products that require no heating, straining, or mixing. The better quality products are alcohol-based liquid extracts or capsules.

The problem with buying these unregulated products, however, is that you cannot be sure what you are getting. Products may or may not contain enough active principle to be effective or they may be contaminated or adulterated with other herbs or ingredients not listed on the label. A report published in the *Los Angeles Times* in 1998 found that only three out of ten brands of St. John's wort contained the amount of the ingredient claimed on the packaging. Commercial herb products are also typically imported from other countries and grown with pesticides and chemicals.

For many of the same reasons people prefer organically grown food, you may want to buy herbs labeled organic or wild crafted. These will not contain pesticide residue and may even be more potent. To find herbs that are grown organically and prepared without alcohol or any animal products (e.g. gelatin), you may need to order them from a specialty mail-order company.

If you prefer making your own remedies from scratch, you can buy herbs that are either whole, cut, or powdered. Powdered herbs will take less time to prepare but don't last as long in storage. You'll need equipment such as a coffee grinder, cheesecloth, mortar, and pestle, etc. (See "At-Home Herbal.")

As with any other medicine, herbs may have adverse effects especially if misused. Therefore:

- Get educated about herbs.
- Use complementary herbs. Sometimes the effect of one herb is too strong. Drawing upon centuries of wisdom, traditional healers use herbs that balance each other's effects for optimum benefit.
- Understand dosage and duration. Certain herbs (e.g. black co-hosh, goldenseal) can be harmful if taken in large doses, and others (kava kava, horsetail) can cause problems if taken over long periods.

- Store herbs safely. You can keep powdered herbs and leaves up to a year; bark for longer. The smell and color of herbs should also tell you whether they have aged and lost effectiveness. Store all herbs in a cool dark place.

Double Trouble? Herb-Drug Interactions

Some herbs and prescription drugs can be a potentially detrimental mix because one enhances the effects of the other, or cancels out the effects. If you are taking any prescription medication, discuss your desire to use herbs with your health care provider. Be sure you understand the effects and side effects of any herb you take before popping over-the-counter medications as well. Examples of herb-drug cocktails to avoid:

Herb	Interacting Drug(s)
Echinacea	Immune suppressants such as prednisone.
Garlic	Anticoagulants (blood thinners) such as Coumadin or aspirin.
Gingko	Anticoagulants (blood thinners) like Coumadin, aspirin, MAO inhibitors such as Nardil, an antidepressant. Antidepressants such as Prozac, Paxil, and Zoloft.
Ginseng	Anticoagulants (blood thinners) such as Coumadin and aspirin.
Kava kava	Sedatives such as Halcion and Valium.
St. John's wort	Antidepressants such as Prozac, Paxil, and Zoloft.

Methods of Application

You can apply herbal therapies in a variety of ways, both externally and internally. The method that will be most effective for you depends on several factors, including the herb, the ailment, and your individual body chemistry. Consult an expert to find out what is best.

Internal

Capsule. This form is best for potent herbs that you need only in small amounts or over a long period. The advantage is convenience and avoidance of the bitter-tasting herbs. You can buy capsules in health food stores and pharmacies; be sure to note the expiration date. To avoid artificial ingredients and fillers, you may want to prepare them at home. To do this, purchase the empty capsules and the herb in powdered form or powder dried herbal extracts yourself in a blender or coffee grinder. Then fill the capsules, packing tightly. Capsule must be stored away from heat and light to preserve potency.

Tea. Medicinal herbal teas prepared at home are superior to commercial brands, which do not typically contain enough active ingredient to be beneficial. When making your own teas, use distilled water or spring water to avoid contaminants. The ratio of dried herb to water is 1 ounce of herb per pint of water; or 2 ounces if you use fresh herbs. Depending on the ailment, the dosage will vary from a few tablespoons a day to a few cups. You may want to prepare many dosages of herbs at once to store for up to three days. Tea types:

• Infusion. This form of a tea is made by first filling a container, such as an enamel teapot, with a pint of just-boiled water and steeping about 2 tablespoons of dried leaves or flowers (more if herbs are fresh) in the water, covered, for up to 20 minutes. You can also use an infuser or tea ball. Strain out herbs before drinking.

• Decoction. This type of tea is made by first chopping or crushing tougher plant parts (coarse leaves, stems, barks, roots) by hand or with a coffee grinder. Boil two ounces of the herbs in a pint of water, then simmer for 20 minutes or up to an hour depending on the herb. Half of the water evaporates during simmering. Strain through a strainer and coffee filter.

Tincture. A concentrated form of herbs, tinctures are best for bitter-tasting or potent herbs or those used over long periods. By combining powdered or cut herbs with alcohol (such as grain alcohol) or glycerin, you can extract the essential ingredients in the herbs and preserve them. Tinctures are widely available in stores, but to make one, add one part chopped or ground herb to two parts alcohol or other solvent in a jar. Cover tightly and store for 4 weeks, shaking daily, then strain. Pour into small bottles using a funnel, label, and store.

Extract. Similar to tinctures, extracts are more concentrated and several times stronger. (See "Oil" below.) The dosage is no more than several drops.

External

Oil. Most frequently made from aromatic herbs such as lavender and rose, oil extracts contain the concentrated power of the essential oils of a given herb. You can buy essential oil preparations in natural food stores and use them in your bath, in a diffuser to spread the scent around your room, or in massage oils. To make your own essential oil extract, ground 2 cups dried or fresh herbs and combine with 4 cups of oil such as olive or sesame oil; let stand in a warm environment or prepare in a double boiler over low heat for an hour. Strain through a strainer lined with a coffee filter; bottle and store. In large doses, essential oils can be irritating—even toxic—so be sure to dilute them before using.

Compress. To prepare this simple but effective method, soak a cloth in an herbal tea, a diluted tincture, or a diluted infused oil. Wring it out, then fold and lay on the affected area of skin. To keep a warm compress warm, resoak or cover with a hot water bottle. Compresses are particularly useful for headaches, menstrual cramps, or muscle or joint pain.

Liniment. Typically used to relieve arthritis or inflammation, a liniment is an herbal preparation that is rubbed into the skin. To prepare, chop fresh or dried herbs finely and place in a jar; add rubbing alcohol until the herbs are covered. Cover and store the herbs for at least 2 weeks, shaking the jar every other day or so. Strain the mixture through a funnel and coffee filter into another jar and label.

Poultice. This herbal preparation is applied to the skin to relieve skin conditions such as bruises or to draw toxins out through the skin. To make a poultice, moisten a powdered herb with hot water, herbal tea, or a tincture. Fold the moistened herbs in gauze then apply it to the affected area. A more old-fashioned way of producing a poultice is to simply chew the fresh herb before applying it to the skin.

Salve. Also applied topically, salves are thick herbal preparations that adhere to the skin to bring about healing. To make a salve, you add one part grated beeswax to four parts infused oil that has been heated to warm. The consistency should be thick, not runny. Pour the salve into a jar, cover, and store. You can also make a salve by adding powdered herbs to hot lard and allow to cool before applying to your skin. To preserve the salve, add benzoin gum or tincture.

Twenty Great Herbs to Have in Your Home

Many herbs are helpful for first aid and minor health problems. Others are useful for preventing or alleviating the symptoms of more serious conditions. According to herbalists, dosages vary depending on the illness and the individual, so check with your practitioner. Herbs for your medicine cabinet include:

Aloe vera *(Aloe vera).* This member of the lily family originated in Africa, where Egyptians used it to soothe wounds. The herb was first commercialized when traders shipped it from Barbados to Europe in the 1600s. Not to be confused with aloe juice, aloe vera gel comes from the center of the aloe plant leaves.

Used to treat: Minor skin irritation, cut, burns. Said to prevent wrinkles.
Parts used: Gel inside leaves.
Application: Gel or liquid.
Caution: Rare allergic reactions. Do not ingest.

Astragalus *(Astragalus membranaceus).* Mainly grown in China, astragalus root has been used in traditional Chinese medicine for centuries.

Used to treat: A general tonic and immune system strengthener. Also for menstrual problems, vaginal infections.
Parts used: Root.
Application: Capsule, tincture.
Caution: None known.

Calendula *(Calendula officinalis).* Believed to have magic powers, calendula has been used by healers since the Dark Ages to soothe the skin.

Used to treat: Skin problems including bruises and burns. Also used to treat ulcers and fevers.
Parts used: Flowers.
Application: Oil, salves, ointments, extracts.
Caution: Do not ingest during pregnancy.

Cat's claw *(Uncaria tomentosa).* Found in the bark of a South American tree, cat's claw is a widely used rainforest herb.

Used to treat: Viral infections, arthritis, irritable bowel.
Parts used: Bark.
Applications: Powder, pills, extracts, tea.
Caution: None known.

Chamomile *(chamomilla recutita).* Two plants share the name and another the properties of this plant that has been called a cure-all.

Used to treat: Insomnia, stress, stomach irritation, digestive disorders, menstrual cramps. May contain antioxidant that fights cancer.

Parts used: Flower.
Applications: Tea, oil, infusion.
Caution: Possible allergic reaction to chamomile pollens.

Dong quai *(Angelica sinensis).* Meaning "proper order," dong quai is an old Chinese remedy that is mentioned in texts dating back to 400 A.D. A similar herb, angelica, is used worldwide for like effects.

Used to treat: Menstrual cramps, irregularity; menopausal symptoms (hot flashes, vaginal dryness); anemia; constipation; and high blood pressure.
Part used: Root.
Applications: Capsule, powder, decoction, tincture.
Cautions: Increased sensitivity to sun is a possible side effect. Do not take dong quai with blood thinners such as coumadin. Do not use during pregnancy.

Echinacea *(Echinacea angustifolia; E. pallida; E. purpurea).* Introduced to a nineteenth-century American doctor by Native American Indians, echinacea was the plant drug of choice to fight infections until the advent of antibiotics in the 1930s.

Used to treat: Colds, flu, respiratory infections. Wounds, urinary tract infections. Stimulates immune system function.
Parts used: Root, leaves.
Application: Tea, tincture, capsules.
Caution: May not be effective after several days of cold/flu; loses effectiveness after 2 weeks. May cause reaction in people with severe eczema. Do not use if you have autoimmune disorder such as lupus or multiple sclerosis.

Evening primrose *(Oenothera biennis).* A New World herb used by Cherokee and Iroquois Indians as food and medicine.

Used to treat: Premenstrual syndrome (PMS), breast pain, meno-

pausal symptoms, inflammatory conditions such as asthma and arthritis. May slow progression of multiple sclerosis. May reverse nerve damage in diabetics.
Parts used: Leaves, seed oil.
Application: Capsule.
Caution: None known.

Feverfew *(Tanacetum parthenium).* Meaning "fever reducer," this aromatic herb was used as far back as 78 A.D.

Used to treat: Headaches/migraines; arthritis.
Parts used: Leaves, flowers.
Applications: Tea, infusion, capsules.
Caution: Mouth sores. Possible stomach upset if used over long periods. Do not use during pregnancy.

Garlic *(Allium sativum).* To ward off illness, Egyptian pyramid workers consumed large amounts of this herb. Originating in the Middle East, garlic is one of the oldest cultivated plants.

Used to treat: High cholesterol, high blood pressure, hardened arteries, heart disease. Infections such as cold and flu.
Parts used: Bulb.
Application: Capsule, powder, oil, freeze-dried tablet, raw herb.
Caution: Too much garlic can cause stomach upset. Clotting problems can result if you also take aspirin or any other anticoagulant (blood thinner).

Ginger *(Zingiber officinale).* Ancient Indian and Chinese healers praised this herb. More than 100,000 tons of this spicy herb are produced each year worldwide. Jamaican ginger is considered the most valuable.

Used to treat: Nausea, morning sickness, motion sickness, upset stomach, diarrhea.
Part used: Root.
Application: Tea, capsule.

Caution: May lower blood pressure excessively in high doses. Consult a health care provider first if you are pregnant or have gallstones.

Ginkgo biloba *(Ginkgo biloba)*. This herb was used by ancient Chinese and Indians for healing and vitality.

Used to treat: Memory, concentration. May improve dementia, Alzheimer's disease, and anxiety. Protects against heart disease.
Parts used: Leaves, nut.
Application: Tablet, capsule, extract.
Caution: Side effects may include headache, allergic reactions, nausea, diarrhea, irritability. Do not take while taking blood thinners such as Coumadin and aspirin.

Ginseng *(Panax ginseng)*. A few different closely related plants carry the name "ginseng." Asian or panax ginseng is a sweet-smelling root long used by Chinese healers. Native Americans turned to American ginseng for a variety of ailments; Siberian ginseng is a close relative. So widely harvested, ginseng has become an endangered species.

Used to treat: Concentration problems, fatigue, stress, sexual dysfunction, aging.
Parts used: Root.
Application: Capsules, extracts.
Caution: Long-term use may cause nervousness, insomnia, headache. Consult a practitioner if you have high blood pressure or diabetes. Avoid if you are pregnant.

Goldenseal *(Hydrastis canadensis)*. The Cherokee Indians first relied on this New World plant to treat skin and eye conditions.

Used to treat: Viral and bacterial infections, colds, flu, sore throats.
Parts used: Root, rhizome.
Application: Tea from root, tincture.

Caution: May cause uterine contractions in pregnant women and raise blood pressure in those with hypertension.

Passionflower *(Passiflora incarnata).* The "passion" part of this herb's name is due to the plants resemblance to Christ's crucifixion, also known as the passion.

Used to treat: Anxiety, nervousness, insomnia, PMS.
Parts used: Flowers, leaves.
Application: Infusion, tincture.
Caution: Consult a practitioner before using in pregnancy.

Red raspberry *(Rubus idaeus).* A common shrub used by Native Americans to ease the pain of childbirth.

Used to treat: Menstrual cramps, endometriosis. Also strengthens uterus during pregnancy and delivery.
Parts used: Leaves, fruit.
Application: Tea, tincture.
Caution: None known.

St. John's wort *(Hypericum perforatum).* This herb is named after St. John the Baptist, whose birthday falls on June 24, during the season when the herb tends to flower. Before its antidepressant qualities became widely known in the United States, many African-Americans used St. John's wort topically for skin conditions.

Used to treat: Anxiety, mild to moderate depression, stomach upset, skin injuries, burns.
Parts used: Leaves, flowering tops.
Application: Tea, powder, capsules, oil.
Caution: Consult a mental health practitioner before taking St. John's wort; serious depression should not be self-treated. High dosage or long-term use of this herb can cause sun sensitivity. Additional side effects may include dry mouth, dizziness, constipation. Look for products that contain hyperforin, the active

ingredient in St. John's wort. Do not combine with other anti-depressants.

Tea tree *(Melaleuca alternifolia)*. New South Wales aborigines used tea tree oil as an antiseptic long before it became a popular home remedy there and throughout the world.

> *Used to treat:* Skin infections.
> *Parts used:* Leaves.
> *Common application:* Oil.
> *Caution:* Possible skin irritation in some people.

Valerian *(Valeriana officinalis)*. Use of valerian root as a sedative dates back to before the Middle Ages. Chinese, Indian, and some European natural healers still use it today.

> *Used to treat:* Sleep disorders including insomnia, nervousness, stress.
> *Parts used:* Rhizome, root.
> *Common applications:* Tea, tincture, tablet, capsule.
> *Caution:* Do not use with other sedatives or alcoholic beverages. Only take before bedtime.

Wild yam *(Dioscorea villosa)*. Also known as rheumatism root for its anti-iflammatory properties, wild yam has become a popular menopausal remedy.

> *Used to treat:* Menstrual cramps, hot flashes, endometriosis, arthritis.
> *Parts used:* Root.
> *Common applications:* Decoction, tincture.
> *Caution:* Possible stomach irritation.

At-Home Herbal: Growing Your Own Medicinal Plants

Whether you have a yard or a pot on your kitchen windowsill, you can grow your own herbs for freshness, purity, convenience, or for the joy of it. These basic tips will help:

1. Plan to create your garden where it will get at least six hours of sunlight each day.
2. Obtain a large bag of ready-to-use organic houseplant soil mix.
3. Obtain plastic, clay, or fiber containers with good drainage holes to prevent root rot.
4. Maximize space by combining several herbs in one container and using hanging baskets.
5. Buy small plants to start, or if you're patient, use seeds. Good choices: basil, parsley, peppermint, rosemary, and sage. Read up on selected herbs to learn growing and usage specifics.
6. Don't overwater, but don't let herbal plants dry out completely.
7. Lightly apply an all-purpose fertilizer by the end of the summer in the first year, and several times each growing season thereafter.
8. When harvesting, pinch or snip plants midmorning when oil content is highest. To prevent molding, be sure plant is dry—no raindrops or dew.
9. To dry, hang upside down by stems inside a paper bag, or place plant parts flat on a screen or wicker tray in a dark, warm, dry, drafty (not damp or humid) place.
10. Label and store in air-tight, opaque containers. Keep in a cool, dark place.

Homeopathy

Meaning "similar" *(homoios)* "suffering" *(pathos)*, homeopathy is based on the idea that a substance that causes symptoms in healthy people can help heal those symptoms in a diseased person. This theory is called the law of similars. Dr. Samuel Hahnemann, the founder of homeopathy, tested this hypothesis on himself and others and discovered that a variety of substances derived from plants, animals, minerals, and chemicals could trigger the body's own healing.

Homeopathy honors the intelligence of the human body. Practitioners see symptoms and disease as the body's response to stress. Instead of suppressing the body's response, homeopathic remedies help *complete* it. Much like herbal remedies, homeopathic remedies act as catalysts, encouraging a physical and psychological response from the body.

Homeopathic remedies are carefully prepared. To avoid worsening a patient's condition, homeopathic remedies are first diluted in alcohol or water, then shaken or *succussed* (ie. struck against the palm to increase potency). This process may be repeated dozens of times. Homeopathic doctors then prescribe remedies based on the individual's symptoms and behavior, not simply on the disease. In this way, homeopathy is truly holistic. Because of the manner in which homeopathy works, you may feel worse before you feel better. Practitioners prescribe remedies for many health challenges, but homeopathy may be particularly effective in treating problems including allergies, headaches, arthritis, and fibromyalgia. Because homeopathy is individualized treatment, it is best to consult a homeopathic healer and not buy generic store brands.

Resources

The American Herbalist Guild, PO Box 70, Roosevelt, UT 84066.

Herb Research Foundation, 1007 Pearl Street, Suite 200, Boulder, CO 80302; *www.herbs.org*

Homeopathy for Women, by Dr. Barry Rose, MRCS, LCRP, DRCOG, FFHom, and Dr. Christina Scott-Moncrieff, MB, ChB, MFHom (Collins + Brown).

Tyler's Honest Herbal, by Steven Foster and Varro E. Tyler, PhD (Haworth Press).

The Way of Herbs, by Micheal Tierra, LAc, OMD (Pocket Books).

The Woman's Book of Healing Herbs, by Sari Harrar and Sara Attshul O'Donnell (Rodale Press).

Chapter 5

❦

Mind-Body Methods

NATURAL WOMAN: MONIQUE FORTUNÉ

During her first experience with meditation, Monique Fortuné could barely control the ticker tape of thoughts running through her mind: I have to write a grocery list, ohmigod, why am I sitting here? Maybe I need to be active. . . . *But gradually, the chatter of her daily to-do list began to quiet down as serenity set in. "My body got still and I said, 'Wait, there is value in being still,'" she recalls.*

A year later, Monique signed up for a meditation workshop with meditation mentor Devya in New York City. She wasn't yet a pro at quieting her mind but she was willing to learn. "At that point in time, I was at a very stressful job," she recalls. "I was a fundraiser and I was also in graduate school. So I felt like I needed to get centered and I needed some peace." During the following year, Monique made the commitment to meditating daily. "I needed to get holistic in my life because I felt that I was running in so many different tracks at one time, I wasn't getting anywhere," she notes. Despite her success as a fundraiser, teacher, radio producer, and community activist, Monique lacked well-being and a sense of her life purpose. Her health was also at stake. Stressed out, she was 50 pounds overweight and her hair was falling out. "I was a good fundraiser," she says. "But I was coming home every day with a headache, sitting in front of the television, eating five pieces of fried chicken, and having a half gallon of ice cream."

Meditation was her balm in Gilead. In mid-1994, she started rising every morning for her meditative practice. Gradually, the stillness and focus she sought began to change her life. "Certain people had to be removed from my life because they were toxic," she says. "Certain situations and people were not serving me. I had to take a hard look at friends, take a hard look at career. Then it took three years later for me to say, 'Oh, your extra weight is not serving you.'" After her morning meditation on June 1, 1997, Monique heard a voice which told her to leave her job.

Three years and a couple of jobs later, the 39-year-old has found her calling: teaching. "I love my students," says the professor of public speaking and philosophy. "Nothing has felt so right." She's also worked with a doctor who helped her to recognize and change her emotional eating patterns. Meditation has put her on and kept her on the correct path. Through deep breathing, meditating on the mantra om, *and praying in front of her altar each day, Monique has discovered the peace of mind and purpose she sought. "The beautiful thing about meditation when you chant [is that] you're feeling that vibration, and when you feel it within you, you feel like you're becoming more whole," she adds.*

When your grandmother said she felt something "in her bones" or that someone "died of a broken heart," she was describing the undeniable link between the mind and the body. Whether we use the term "mind-body," "mind, body, spirit," or the more inclusive "mind, body, spirit, and emotions," we are describing the truly whole and integrated nature of ourselves, of our beings. Whereas Western medicine has separated the mind and the body, and largely ignored the importance of mental and spiritual health up until recently, Eastern healers have long recognized the interconnectedness of the parts that make up the whole. Indeed, many traditional healers believe that illness or "dis-ease" begins in our minds, with an emotion, and manifests in the body as symptoms. Mind-body medicine is based at least in part on the idea that to heal a physical illness, we must first address the underlying emotional or spiritual cause.

Science is beginning to take notice. Recently a new field of medicine known as psychoneuroimmunology has emerged to specifically study the interplay between the mind and the nervous and immune systems. Researchers at the University of Rochester have actually measured the effect of emotional stress on the duration of a cold, for example. Experts in this area have also demonstrated how relaxation techniques can lower blood pressure. A study published in the journal *Hypertension* in 1996 found that by practicing Transcendental Meditation (TM) over a period of three months, older African-Americans were able to significantly lower their blood pressure. This was true even for those who were at high risk for hypertension because of stress, obesity, alcohol use, physical inactivity, and high sodium intake.

Mind-body methods, ranging from support groups, meditation, and guided imagery to yoga and spiritual healing have been used successfully to help treat problems as diverse as heart disease, high cholesterol, cancer, diabetes, and arthritis, according to the National Center for Complementary and Alternative Medicine of the National Institutes of Health. This is a fact that black women have long understood, if only intuitively. By saying a prayer generations ago or joining a sister circle today, we've been workin' some of the most powerful and now proven mind-body therapies.

Natural Healing Is Our Heritage

To our West African ancestors, the mind-body-spirit connection was unquestionable. It is the basis of the African worldview. As Malidome Somé writes in *The Healing Wisdom of Africa*: "A physical body alone cannot have any sort of direction in this life, so it is important to recognize that the body is an extension of the spirit, and the spirit is an extension of the body, and that the two are inseparable, with a communication that goes both ways." Because the body and spirit are one, illness is not only the result of physical symptoms, but an underlying "energetic" or spiritual disorder, Somé explains. The cure, therefore, has to address the spiritual level in order to be effective and enduring. In the Dagara village where Somé was trained in the ways of a shaman, and in many indigenous African communities, deep healing does not rely first and foremost on a pill or medical treatment, but on consultation with elders and ancestors, and on a return to nature, ritual, and community. "Healing," he notes, "comes when the individual remembers his or her identity . . . and reconnects with that world of Spirit."

This world of Spirit includes our ancestors, spirits, or inanimate objects imbued with spiritual power. Nature is the magical home of these other-worldly beings, the point of contact. Though unseen, these ancestors and spirits are always present, offering guidance and wisdom when it is needed. For Africans, the interconnectedness of the body, mind, and spirit, therefore, is not limited to the individual person but it extends also to the family, community, ancestors, nature, and the universe.

For African-Americans this strong relationship with Spirit has survived though in different forms. Stripped of the freedom to practice their beliefs openly, our enslaved ancestors embraced Christianity while also holding fast to faith in the power of "spirits," ancestors, and even hexes created by those who worked "roots." In Toni Morrison's *Beloved,* we witness both the belief in a vengeful spirit in the form of Beloved as well as the power of prayer to conquer the devil-child's power and restore Sethe to health.

Today black women dominate the pews in black churches and some are wielding the reigns of power in the pulpits. More and more sisters follow Islam, Yoruba, and other African religions. Still others embrace New Age spirituality. In many ways, black women's reliance on prayer—whether it is to God, Allah, a Higher Power, or Mother Spirit—has always superseded a reliance on the tools of Western medicine. Perhaps this is due to ancient wisdom that we still carry within us.

This Far by Faith

Black women have longed believed in prayer's power to bring about a healing. Among sisters, praying for the sick is not considered a last, desperate resort, but a first course of treatment as important as conventional Western remedies. This belief was borne out in the life of Reverend Dr. Barbara King, who healed from the physical challenge of tuberculosis by repeating several times daily a prayer that contained the potent words, "God is my health; I can't be sick."

Researchers have found that patients feel better and get well sooner when they either attend religious services, pray for themselves, or get prayed for. The most astonishing studies have shown improvements among patients who did not even know others were praying for them. The key, from the standpoint of researchers, lies not in a particular religious affiliation or prayer, but in the sense of comfort people gain from their spirituality. Praying can help us manage stress, experts say. "It keeps you sane," says Denese Shervington, MD, MPH, a psychiatrist and author of *Soul Quest: A Healing Journey for Women of the African Diaspora*. "It allows you to tolerate and accept the ebb and flow of life." Joining religious institutions can also eliminate isolation and provide us with the support we need to take the very best care of ourselves.

From the standpoint of mind-body practitioners, faith in a healing power greater than ourselves works in part because our beliefs affect our reality; in fact, they *are* our reality. As Jesus said to the sick woman who had touched his garments from behind, "Daughter, your faith has made you well; go in peace, and be healed of your disease."

How to Tap into the Power of Spiritual Healing

- Say a little prayer. Many of us learned to pray by asking God/Spirit for what we don't have. Another way is to thank God/Spirit for *what is,* to affirm that we've already been given all that we need.

- Hook up with a prayer circle or group. Tara Harper of New York is a member of a group that stops to pray at noon each day.
- Join a spiritual community. This may or may not be a church or mosque, but it should be a group of people on a spiritual path that mirrors your own.

Relaxation Techniques

"Relaaaax!" says a loving friend, partner, or health care provider to us, but that is often easier said than done. It may be safe to say that many black women simply don't know how to relax. We've been focusing on making it and taking care of others for so long, we feel guilty even thinking about relaxation. But taking a break and putting our minds at ease is no luxury to be indulged during annual vacations; it is a health necessity. When we actively engage in relaxation techniques such as meditation or yoga, we naturally slow our brain waves, relax our muscles, and allow the power of mind-body healing to come forward.

The beauty of the following techniques is that you can do them by yourself at any time and in any place. Ten to twenty minutes should be enough time to trigger the relaxation response in your body, but you may want to add more over time to maximize the healing benefits. Try to incorporate these relaxation techniques into your morning and evening routines. When we are most stressed or in despair, a relaxation technique may be the last thing we feel like doing, but it may be what we most need to do. If one technique does not seem to work for you, try another until you find one that fits.

Meditation

Focused awareness is one way to describe meditation, an ancient Eastern spiritual practice. "It's a way of calming the thought waves of your mind," says Devya, a New York City meditation mentor and president of Devya and Associates. "Meditation gives you a period of time where the thoughts quiet down so that you can begin to tap into the real wisdom that lies within you."

Your meditation can take many forms. You can begin by finding a quiet spot to sit comfortably in the cross-legged half-lotus position with hands resting, palms facing up or down, on your knees. Or if that is uncomfortable or distracting for you, try sitting upright in a chair with hands resting on (not clutching) your knees, or lying down on your back with arms at your sides, palms open. Close your eyes. Notice your breathing. If a thought enters your mind, observe it and let it go.

For beginners, Devya suggests simply breathing from the diaphragm and counting to ten: *One*, breathe in and out; *two*, inhale, exhale, and so on. If you lose count, start over. This builds concentration. Another technique, called even breathing, involves breathing in to a count of *one, two, three, four*, and breathing out, *one, two, three, four*. Devya recommends meditating twice a day for twenty minutes but once a day is sufficient for relaxation.

If you have difficulty concentrating and becoming relaxed, take a meditation course at your local Y, a gym, or a yoga center. Some churches even offer meditation instruction. Also consider buying relaxation tapes.

NATURAL WOMAN: TERESA WILTZ

Thirty-eight-year-old writer Teresa Wiltz first got into meditation several years ago to "find some peace" during a particularly stressful period of her life. Now her daily practice is as spiritual as it is relaxing. "It's more a spiritual practice and the by-product is that I'm more centered and grounded," she says.

After showering and stretching each morning, Teresa lights a candle, burns some incense, and sits to read from inspirational books. After a few minutes, she either chants mantras like oom *or performs breathing techniques until she experiences a deep stillness. "I get into this deep trance feeling which is just pure bliss," she says. Meditation has helped Teresa not only to overcome the anxieties of life and a profession run by deadlines, but also to develop self-trust and her connection to Spirit. "I believe in God now because I meditate, because of what I feel," she adds.*

Meditation takes time to learn. You may want to experiment with different techniques to reap the profound mental, physical, and spiritual benefits of meditation. To reach this rejuvenating state of altered awareness, experiment with the methods described below. Begin with ten minutes once or twice a day and work up to twenty minutes.

Breathing. With eyes shut, inhale slowly. Picture the air moving through your body toward your toes. After a pause, exhale and see the air flowing away from you. Concentrate on the expansion and contraction of your abdomen with each breath.

Chanting. A Hindu practice introduced to the West in the 1960s, Transcendental Meditation popularized mantra meditation, a method in which a word or phrase is continually repeated, silently or aloud. Close your eyes and chant the Hindi *Om* or *Peace* or *I am strong* each time you exhale.

Gazing. Without thinking about it in words, watch a candle flame, a flower, or another object a foot away from you. Keep your breathing steady as you free your mind of everything else. If your mind or gaze wanders, gently return to the object.

Visualization. Close your eyes and picture the tension seeping out of every muscle, from head to toe, as you exhale. Noting each detail, see yourself on a deserted beach, in a quiet garden, or in another calm locale.

Emptying your mind. With eyes open or closed, focus on letting all thoughts float by as if meaningless.

Breath Work

Concentrating on and controlling our breathing is one basic way to immediately focus the mind and relax our spirits. Breath work can also increase the amount of oxygen flowing through the body and enhance our energy.

Breathe Awareness. To perform this breathing technique, simply concentrate on the feel and sound of your breath moving in and out of your body. Don't try to force a change in your breathing pattern at first; just observe. After several minutes have passed, make an effort to breathe more fully, filling the abdomen, then the chest as you inhale; empty the chest and abdomen as you exhale. Slow your breathing down, taking more time to exhale than inhale.

Square Breathing. If breathe awareness proves difficult, breathe in slowly for four counts, hold for four, then breathe out for four. Repeat the cycle several times until you feel your breath is under your control.

Alternate Nostril Breathing. When you feel comfortable controlling your breath, try this technique: Empty your lungs. With a hand placed lightly over your nose, close your left nostril and breathe in through the right nostril for six to eight counts. Close the right nostril and hold your breath for four counts. Open the left nostril and breathe out for six to eight counts. Breathe in through the left nostril, then close it for four counts, and breathe out through the right nostril. Repeat this cycle until you are completely relaxed. You may even feel light-headed.

Progressive Muscle Relaxation

This form of relaxation is particularly helpful for easing tension stored in the head, neck, or shoulders. Begin by lying down, preferably on the floor with legs parted, arms loosely at your sides. Tense your toes for a few seconds and release them. Then work upward from your feet, thighs, and buttocks to your stomach, hands, arms, neck, and face. Take your time as you isolate each muscle, including your jaw, eyes, and forehead. Lie quietly when you are done.

Mind over Matter

Some effective mind-body techniques require the help of others, at least at first. In addition to quieting the mind, we can focus it on what we want it to do. These include:

Guided Imagery or Visualization

If picturing clear blue ocean water or a green pasture brings you a sense of peace, you know what guided imagery is about. Through guided imagery, we bring to mind an image that can facilitate healing in the body. But this is not a passive daydream: Imagery or visualization is active imagining which includes all of your senses. We often waste a lot of time imagining the worst in our lives—that we'll arrive late to some important appointment or that someone will let us down. Guided imagery uses the same mental power in a positive way.

Many athletes use imagery to visualize themselves performing the perfect vault or jump. The same technique can be applied to healing. You can use guided imagery after meditation or a breathing exercise, when you are feeling relaxed and open. You may simply want to visualize yourself in perfect health and at peace. Or you might try visualizing the shrinking of a fibroid tumor, for example. Do this for fifteen to twenty minutes several times a week or every day to achieve the desired result.

Tara Harper uses visualizations to make the most of each day. "If something important is going on that day, I visualize how that's going to go," she explains. "And then I visualize long-term goals. I believe that if you act according to your visualization, as if it were already completed, then it gets completed." In studies, researchers have found that patients using guided imagery reduced levels of cortisol, a potent stress hormone, in the blood. Visualization can also help women coping with breast cancer treatment. Studies have also shown positive effects with colon cancer, multiple sclerosis, bulimia, posttraumatic stress disorder, pain, and anxiety.

Hypnotherapy

Also known as hypnosis, hypnotherapy is a technique that uses the power of suggestion to heal. While in a state of focused relaxation, you may be more open to ideas that help you relinquish a fear or an addiction, for example. Hypnosis, which means "sleep," is not a state in which others control you, but one in which you can reach a deeper state of consciousness with the help of a licensed hypnotherapist or other facilitator.

How does hypnosis work? A psychotherapist, nurse, dentist, or other licensed professional trained in hypnotherapy will help bring you to this concentrated state by counting or repeating a word. While you are in this trancelike condition, the hypnotist can use suggestion, imagery, and other techniques to help you relieve stress, pain, and other ailments. A hypnotherapist can also teach you to hypnotize yourself.

Hypnotherapy works best if you are open to it and really ready to change a negative behavior. It has been shown to help with conditions such as obesity, irritable bowel syndrome, cancer, multiple sclerosis, headache, anxiety associated with dental treatments, and pain. To locate a hypnotherapist, see the Resources.

Biofeedback

This mind-body technique shows you how to control functions of the body that are normally automatic such as breathing, blood pressure, muscle tension, and skin temperature. By controlling these functions, you can learn to relax the body at will and alleviate various health problems.

Depending on the condition you are trying to heal, a therapist will hook you up to a biofeedback machine that measures either brain waves, breathing, sweat, muscle tension, pulse, or temperature. The feedback from the machine will show you how you can change your body's reactions by changing your thoughts. With time and practice, you should be able to relax your body functions without the machine.

How can biofeedback help you? In addition to giving you a tool to relieve stress, biofeedback may alleviate symptoms of asthma, hypertension, headache, incontinence, stroke, and addiction, among others.

Mental Health Help

Psychotherapy

Though many of us used to think of psychotherapy as something for white folks, more sisters are turning to mental health services and more black therapists are available to guide us in reclaiming our emotional health. Black women are not immune to depression and suicide as we were so painfully reminded when singer Phyllis Hyman committed suicide in 1995, an apparent victim of chronic loneliness. In fact, research has indicated that black women are more prone to depression than white women, though the condition may manifest in different ways in us (e.g., weight gain, chronic fatigue). Considering our higher rates of fatherlessness, and sexual and physical abuse—coupled with the impact of both racism and sexism—it should come as no surprise that a National Center for Health Statistics study comparing the mental health of various groups identified sisters as the unhappiest group in America.

We can no longer afford to neglect our emotional well-being. Psychotherapists can, of course, help you through a crisis such as a sudden loss of a loved one, divorce, rape or trauma. But there are many other benefits as well. In psychotherapy, you can gain a clearer understanding of your behavior, and learn concrete coping strategies. A psychotherapist can help you uncover the roots of low self-esteem, anxiety, addictive behavior and depression. The therapist is not there to tell you what to do, as many folks believe, but to support you in your emotional growth and healing. If you are hesitant to seek the help of a "shrink," try to think of the practitioner as just one of the many "guides" and advice givers in your life. Remind yourself that asking for help is *not* a sign of weakness but of maturity and strength. Asking for help may go against your superwoman tendencies—the desire to take on and do too much at work, at home, and in the community, to prove we can do it all and look good too. Therapy can help us break this self-destructive pattern.

Depending on the depth of your emotional challenge and your commitment to getting better, psychotherapy may take as little as a few weeks to several months or years to be effective. Regardless of how long it might take, if you are feeling blue (e.g. lack of interest in activities you once enjoyed, thoughts of worthlessness—see signs of depression in Chapter 14) for more than a couple of weeks, make an appointment with a qualified therapist. Ask friends and family members for referrals. You may want to schedule a consultation first to see if you feel at ease with the therapist. You may prefer a woman or a black woman who can understand the unique pressures of being female and of African descent. Some forms of psychotherapy will simply involve "talk," and others will require some homework on your part. (See "Ask an Expert.")

Spiritual Counseling

The blending of mental health counseling with spirituality is becoming more common and is appealing to us as a spiritual people. In this type of counseling, you and the practitioner can draw upon the tools of psychology and faith to bring about healing. A spiritual counselor may be a psychologist, psychotherapist, psychiatrist, or social worker on a spiritual path, or a minister or pastoral counselor with mental health training. This type of counseling recognizes that we are as much spiritual beings as mental and emotional ones. If your religious faith or spirituality is a vital part of your life, you may want a counselor who affirms and respects your beliefs.

Much like psychotherapy, spiritual counseling is designed to help you understand yourself and the problem and to learn coping strategies with an emphasis on faith as part of the solution. This does not mean that prayer alone will cure depression or addiction. It is a complement to the inner work you may need to do with the help of a trained professional. To find a spiritual counselor, ask for referrals from people you know and check your local church or other religious institution.

Additional Mental Health Therapies

Group Therapy. This alternative to one-on-one therapy provides the advantage of group support and interaction. Many psychotherapists and other mental health practitioners offer this option in their practice.

Twelve-step groups. A type of group therapy, twelve-step groups, such as Alcoholic Anonymous, are structured programs that help people break addictions, including drinking, drugs, gambling, and overeating.

Gestalt Therapy. This creative form of therapy involves various techniques—role playing, visualization, creative expression—in addition to talk therapy. This holistic approach offers many tools to increase self-knowledge and behavioral change.

Re-birthing. This therapy is based on the belief that expressing traumas experienced early in life clears emotional blocks and facilitates healing. Using a technique called conscious-connected breathing, a re-birthing therapist helps you relive and release emotionally troubling experiences—even the trauma of birth.

Art Therapy. Making art came quite naturally to all of us as children. Whether you consider yourself an artist or not today, art therapy is an effective tool for relieving tension and stress, and even deeper emotional problems. You can indulge in this therapy by drawing or making a collage on your own, or by finding an art therapist at a local hospital or art school.

Music Therapy. Listening to soothing music can be good medicine. For stress, Wendy Webb swears by gospel music. "Best cure there is!" she notes. Making music is also therapeutic whether you can carry a tune or play an instrument. "When you make certain tones and sing certain words, they communicate to your body," says Ayesha Grice, who writes and performs her own songs for pleasure and stress relief.

Pet Therapy. Research shows that older folks who live with pets live longer than those who live alone. For this reason, some hospitals and nursing homes regularly provide pets for patients to stroke and cuddle with. A loyal dog, cat, or hamster provides companionship, unconditional love—and a way to ease stress.

Ask an Expert

A number of different mental health experts are trained to help you with emotional challenges. To find a good practitioner, start by asking friends or relatives for referrals. Some of these providers will charge fees on a sliding scale basis. Here's a breakdown of the types of experts you might find and their training.

Psychotherapists, who can be psychiatrists, psychologists, or social workers, use talking therapy to solve emotional problems. Depending on the rules in the state you live in, unlicensed practitioners can also call themselves psychotherapists, so ask about training during an initial phone call or consultation.

Psychiatrists are physicians (MDs) who have undergone additional training in diagnosing and treating mental disorders and emotional problems. They can prescribe medication.

Psychologists who have doctoral degrees (PhDs, EdDs, or PsyDs) in human psychology. They may be trained in various therapies and some specialize in marriage and family therapy.

Social workers usually have master's or doctoral degrees (MSWs, CSWs, or DSWs). Often from a community activist perspective, they counsel people on life issues from substance abuse and domestic violence to nutrition and housing.

Certified pastoral counselors bring a spiritual perspective to therapy and must have at least a master's of divinity degree (MDiv).

Self-Help

Support Groups

Sometimes nothing beats getting together with some girlfriends to discuss a book, to organize around community issues, or to talk "man" problems. And many black women are using sister support networks to cope with health issues of all kinds—from lupus to hirsutism to sarcoidosis to cancer. The sister circle trend has evolved into a movement, helping women to first take refuge then turn around and take charge of their lives. In these informal groups, black women find affirmation, friendship, information, encouragement, and social support—a factor that scientific researchers are finding is critical for health and well-being.

Studies have found that women with breast cancer increase their chance of survival when they receive support either in groups or one-on-one. One small study also found that diabetics who were in support groups were better able to control blood sugar. In a well-known program to reverse heart disease, support groups are as important an element as a low-fat diet and exercise. The experts believe this is because support from others serves as a buffer against stress. Support may also boost our immune response. The encouragement of others motivates us to take the very best care of ourselves as well. Hafeezah, a New York City consultant and founder of A Circle of Sisters, sees additional benefits. "Women recognize that they are not alone," she says. Support groups bring us out of our isolation and back into the community that our ancestors relied on for healing. "What we're longing for is to be with other people of like mind," she notes.

The National Black Women's Health Project has been helping women to organize around health issues since 1983, and its support groups can be found nationwide. You can join or start your own groups by word of mouth, by inquiring at a local hospital or clinic, or by advertising in local newspapers. Sister support groups typically have no leader, are small enough in number for each member to have a chance to talk, and meet regularly—at least once a month.

Any additional rules can be set by the group and changed if need be. Your goal is to *be there* for yourselves and for each other in a non-judgmental and loving environment—to listen, provide encouragement, and share success strategies without giving advice. You can also incorporate other mind-body healing techniques, such as prayer, in your group.

Affirmative Attitude

If you look through the black section of your local bookstore, among the history books and autobiographies, you'll find several books of affirmations. What are these words exactly? "Affirmations are essentially a conscious, intentional, judicious use of words for self-talk," says Andriette Earl-Bozeman, a spiritual counselor, coach, and workshop facilitator in Oakland, California. The idea is that because we are always doing some form of self-talk (anything from *"I look fat!"* to *"I'm going to make a wonderful presentation today."*), we might as well make the majority of those thoughts positive. "I would say bottom line is to train the mind," Earl-Bozeman explains. "The mind is so powerful and most of us have trained it unconsciously. That is to say it's been trained by television, commercial radio. So it's not that anyone has an untrained mind. It's just that it has not been trained consciously and intentionally with a positive result in mind."

Black women especially may benefit from this form of positive thinking, says Earl-Bozemnan, because so much of our "training" has been the result of negative stereotyping.

Self-Awareness Tool

What Are You Thinking?

Pick a day this week to get a handle on your thoughts. You may be surprised by how many negative ideas and beliefs run through your mind—and run your life and health. Make a point from the beginning of the day to the end to jot down in a notebook, day planner, or this book every cynical or self-defeating notion you come up with. A few examples: *I messed up again! I never get anything right. I'm a failure.* Or your thoughts might sound more like *S/he doesn't like me. He's out to get me. Life is too hard.* Make note of your thoughts here:

_____

_____

_____

_____

_____

Once you've written your negative thoughts down, take a good look at them. Are they *really* true? Try coming up with evidence to the contrary. This awareness and reframing should help diffuse the tyranny of negative thoughts in your mind, or help you brainstorm ways to change a negative situation.

Journaling

You don't have to be a writer to benefit from putting your thoughts on paper. One recent study showed that a group of asthmatics suffered fewer symptoms after they were asked to write about a traumatic experience in their lives. Journaling is a form of emotional release and it is as simple as putting pen to paper. You can write simple words, a paragraph, or pages of your thoughts at the beginning or end of each day. These need not be well-written entries but they should be from your heart—unedited. You can write to record your experiences or simply to get thoughts out of your head. You can write to yourself, to God, to an ancestor, or to no one at all. Over time, you can return to your journal entries to note progression in your healing and to learn from your experiences. Let your journaling time be your time.

Resources

Academy for Guided Imagery, PO Box 2070, Mill Valley, CA 94942.

American Council of Hypnotist Examiners, 700 S. Central Avenue, Glendale, CA 91204.

American Society of Clinical Hypnosis, 33 West Grand Avenue, Suite 402, Chicago, IL 60610.

Association for Applied Psychophysiology and Biofeedback, 10200 W. Forty-fourth Avenue, Suite 304, Wheat Ridge, CO 80033-2840.

Center for Mind-Body Medicine, 5225 Connecticut Avenue, NW, Suite 414, Washington, D.C., 20015.

Insight Meditation Society, 1230 Pleasant Street, Barre, MA 01005.

Mind/Body Medical Institute, 110 Francis Street, Ste. 1A, Boston, MA 02215.

In the Spirit, by Susan L. Taylor (Harper Collins).

Lessons in Living, by Susan L. Taylor (Doubleday).

Soul Quest: A Healing Journey for Women of the African Diaspora, by Denese Shervington, MD, MPH, and Billie Jean Pace, MD (Random House).

Transform Your Life, by Rev. Dr. Barbara King (Berkley).

Chapter 6

⟡

Laying On of Hands

A back injury sent Carol (who asked not to use her real name) first to a massage therapist and then to a chiropractor in spring 1999. She'd gone horseback riding and felt a peculiar sensation in her spine. At that point in her life, Carol was no stranger to doctors. Since she had dislocated her hip while running at age 14 and had to have her spleen removed, she'd suffered a number of health problems including heavy bleeding and severe cramping during menstruation. Over the years the 34-year-old freelance writer and videographer has been diagnosed with everything from hyperglycemia and hypoglycemia to connective tissue disorder. "All of my systems were basically breaking down," she recalls.

After experimenting with a special diet and supplements for several months, Carol's riding accident sent her to the healer who could finally help her. At the chiropractic office of Dr. Alfred Davis, Jr., in Monclair, New Jersey, Carol received daily spinal adjustments for two weeks. She also began taking supplements for her multiple health challenges. After two weeks, she noticed the severe menstrual cramping she was so used to was subsiding. Within two months, "I noticed that I wasn't as fatigued, that I didn't have to rest during the day," says the woman who had switched to working from home because of her physical state. "I had a lot more energy than before." In addition to the less frequent but continued chiropractic treatments, Carol began exercising for a half hour each day.

Carol learned that because of misalignments in her spine that originated when she was still a teenager, nerves that influenced other systems in her body had been affected. Once the spinal problems were addressed, her symptoms improved. These days, she visits the chiropractor once every two to three weeks. After years of searching for answers to her mysterious ailments, Carol feels fine.

Hands-On Healing

The reassuring pleasure of a warm hug or pat on the back are just hints of the power that human touch has to heal and restore us. In the previous chapter you learned about how the mind can be focused and applied to bring about healing; this chapter deals with natural healing techniques that utilize the hands and other noninvasive instruments and tools to heal. In some cases, such as chiropractic or massage, a practitioner uses the hands to manipulate or stimulate the physical body. In others, such as acupuncture and the laying on of hands, the practitioner's hands serve as channels of universal energy flowing through the body. Either way, hands-on healing assists the body in restoring itself to balance and well-being.

Though scientists were once doubtful of these methods, in recent years sound research has shown the effectiveness of such therapies as chiropractic, acupuncture, and massage. In 1997, an expert panel organized by the National Institutes of Health concluded that acupuncture alone was effective in treating postoperative and chemotherapy nausea and postoperative dental pain. As an adjunct to other therapies, acupuncture was found to be useful for people with health challenges such as headache, menstrual cramps, asthma, fibromyalgia, and low back pain. Experts have also recently recognized that chiropractic—long ridiculed by Western medicine—is an effective backache treatment. Studies also point to several therapeutic uses for massage. Maybe that is why, after allopathic medicine, massage and chiropractic are the two largest health care systems in the United States.

Natural Healing Is Our History

Though our African ancestors did not practice such forms of hands-on healing as acupuncture, they did believe in the notion of an invisible "energy" running through the body, and through all living things, that is similar to the *qi* or "chi" recognized in traditional Chinese medicine. According to West African healer Malidoma Patrice Somé, this energy, too, could become blocked, causing illness. In *The Healing Wisdom of Africa,* he says, "all healing must begin by first addressing the energetic problems," which originate in the mind and spirit.

Our ancestors were among the first to practice many hands-on therapies. "Egyptians massaged their warriors before they [went off] to war so they'd be prepared," says Renee Wiggins, founder of Results by Renee, a practice that offers personal training, nutrition consultation, and massage in Silver Springs, Maryland. "Then they massaged them when they got back because of the injuries they sustained."

Healing with Touch

Touch is perhaps the oldest form of healing, dating back to a time when human beings had no drugs or instruments other than human hands. Over the centuries, practitioners have perfected various types of healing that involve touch and the manipulation of different body parts including the muscles, neck, and spine. The goal of all of these hands-on methods is to correct imbalances that cause discomfort and disease.

However, many of us have lost touch—no pun intended—with the value of touch and are either uncomfortable with it or suspicious of it. "I find that some black women never had a stranger touch them before," says Wiggins. " A lot of them think of it as being sexual." In those cases, she reminds sisters that massage is therapeutic and nurturing. "What did our mothers do when we were sick or in tears?" she asks. "[They] rubbed us, held us. And we always felt that made the pain go away." But Wiggins also acknowledges that some women may shy away from touch therapy because of a history of physical or sexual abuse. These survivors can be reintroduced to touch in non-threatening ways through massage and other hands-on healing methods.

The major touch therapies that involve the manipulation of the body to correct imbalances include:

Chiropractic

Meaning "done by hand," chiropractic is one of the most popular forms of alternative healing in the United States. Today, the majority of private insurers and HMOs that serve large employers cover chiropractic care. Chiropractors believe that because all nerve impulses pass from the brain through the spine to the rest of the body, spinal misalignments can impede vital communication between the brain and the body. This interference, or subluxation as chiropractors call it, may be caused by poor posture, physical traumas, or injuries. It can result in tension and poor blood flow. "The basic principle of chiropractic is that the brain sends electrical information down the spinal cord," says Alfred Davis, Jr., of Davis Chiropractic Center in Montclair, New Jersey. "That information exits out via spinal nerves from the spinal column and those nerves go to each and every cell of the body either directly or indirectly. So all the functionings of the systems, glands, organs, muscles, and ligaments are controlled by the nervous system."

To treat subluxation and restore balance to the body, chiropractors make adjustments, or gentle thrusts with their hands that realign the vertebrae. They may do this while you are sitting up or lying down in various positions. In some cases, patients reexperience an old trauma or pain of a physical or emotional nature. Releasing this pain may cause discomfort initially followed by total body healing.

Chiropractic is best known for its effectiveness in treating back pain but it can also help heal neck pain, sciatica (inflammation of the sciatic nerve), headaches, and arthritis. The founder of chiropractic in this country, Daniel David Palmer, restored hearing to a deaf patient using this method in 1895. Dr. Davis has helped patients relieve symptoms of premenstrual syndrome, menopause—and even helped some women get pregnant by correcting misalignments in the pelvis. Today some chiropractors incorporate other natural healing modalities such as nutrition, massage, physical therapy and ultrasound electrical stimulation in their practice. When you enter a chiropractor's office, the practitioner will take a history, check vital signs, assess your spine and nerve health, and determine if chiropractic is for you. An initial session should take at least about a half hour. Depending on the severity of the problem, your symptoms may subside after just one treatment or several. Dr. Davis believes everyone should get their spine checked, and he generally recommends that clients return for an evaluation once a month.

Massage

Also known as massage therapy, this form of health care involves the manipulation of muscles and soft tissue to promote relaxation and well-being. The manual stimulation of skin, tissue, and nerves has endless benefits: improved blood and lymph flow, enhanced nutrition of tissues, reduced inflammation, quickened waste removal, and pain relief. Of course, massage is very relaxing and it can actually lower blood pressure within minutes. Massage generally has no negative effects but you should avoid it you are menstruating heavily, or have a blood clot (because massage can stimulate bleeding or swelling), fever, or broken skin.

Massage therapy has evolved over centuries into a practice that is used by many different cultures in different ways. From the ancient Chinese system of massage, therapists worldwide have created dozens of various techniques which have different benefits, including those designed for pregnant women and survivors of physical or emotional abuse. If you have a history of physical or sexual abuse, any form of touch therapy may feel uncomfortable or seem threatening. But some massage therapists are trained to help you. To increase your comfort level, you may also want to seek out a therapist of color to treat you. In that case, ask your friends, relations, and health care provider for referrals. It may take some footwork but the increased sense of comfort may be worth it. Many massage therapists combine more than one technique to maximize the benefits to the client. To find a qualified massage therapist, ask for referrals from friends and your health care provider. Common massage styles include:

Swedish Massage. Named for a Swedish practitioner who combined Chinese massage methods with Western science, this style is probably the most well known and widely used in the United States. Swedish massage therapists use five basic strokes (effleurage, petrissage, friction, tapotement, and vibration) to improve muscle tone and increase circulation. In a typical session, you lie down on a massage table while the practitioner works methodically on your different body parts using massage oil as a lubricant. With her or his hands, the therapist can assess the condition of underlying tissue and apply pressure where it is needed. Depending on your preference, you can make an appointment for a half-hour massage or one as long as an hour and a half.

Deep Tissue Massage. A more intense form of hands-on therapy than Swedish massage, deep tissue massage or deep tissue therapy presses more deeply into the muscles and connective tissue to alleviate tension and pain. A practitioner will focus more specifically on tender spots, applying deep strokes to initiate healing. You may feel discomfort during and after this type of massage before you feel better. Deep tissue massage is particularly helpful for chronic pain or injuries, but it is also good for general health maintenance.

Sports Massage. This specialized massage form was developed to help athletes, dancers, and others who frequently tax their muscles to recover from injury, muscle fatigue, and pain. The sports massage therapist uses specific strokes (trigger point pressure, cross-fiber friction and compression) to increase circulation to any sensitive area, improve flexibility, stimulate muscles, and assist waste removal. Performed before or after workouts or competitions, sports massage minimizes the risk of injury. This rigorous massage therapy may be combined with hydrotherapy (see below) and ice packs to reduce swelling. A session can last anywhere from 15 minutes to an hour.

Medical Massage. Much like Swedish massage, medical massage utilizes specific strokes for rehabilitation or the treatment of a number of illnesses. The strokes are designed to increase circulation, nourish tissues, and promote flexibility and healing. A medical massage therapist will work specifically on an affected area or system for about a half hour.

Osteopathy

Once referred to as "bone setters," modern osteopaths derive their title from words meaning "bone" *(osteo)* and "suffer" *(pathic)*. Their healing system, osteopathic manipulative medicine (OMM), focuses primarily on the health of the musculoskeletal system in order to maintain health of the entire body. Much like chiropractors, osteophathic physicians (DOs) administer hands-on manipulations to maintain proper structure and functioning of the body. This in turn strengthens the immune system and overall well-being. Once you are examined by an osteopathic physician, you receive a manipulation once or twice a week depending on the problem. These manipulations may consist of mild twists or more forceful thrusts to the back, arms, legs, or head. Different techniques are applied to release energy, promote blood and lymph circulation, and restore full range of motion.

The manipulation, called osteopathic manipulative treatment (OMT), can help improve posture and alleviate back and neck pain, headaches, and arthritis. Osteopaths can also advise you on nutrition, exercise, and prevention. Some even offer acupuncture, massage, and other techniques. Classical osteopathy was and is a drugless medicine. But because many conventional osteopaths are now trained like medical doctors, they can also administer standard medical examinations and tests, as well as medication and surgery, if needed.

Reflexology

According to reflexologists, a good foot rub is more than just that. Reflexology is another ancient healing system practiced by African healers. Njideka N. Olatunde, ND, PhD, founder of Focus on Healing Wellness Services in Washington, D.C., explains that Egyptian art depicts black healers working on the feet and hands of others. "Reflexology is over 5,000 years old," says Olatunde. "The first tools man ever had in terms of healing were their hands. By using the hands in reflexology, we were able to design a technique that has spread all across the world.

"Reflexology is the art and science of working specific reflex and pressure point areas on the hands, feet, and ears to relax and release stress, pain, and discomfort," she says. Reflexologists believe that by applying pressure to specific points in the foot, which correspond to specific organs and glands, a practitioner can stimulate nerves, blood flow, and healing. "All nerve endings, which are connected to the specific systems and organs in the body, end in the hands and feet," Olatunde explains. "So you can activate systems and organs through the hands, feet, and ears." Using just their hands, reflexologists work on one part of the body—namely the soles of the feet, palms of the hands, or ears—in order to bring balance to others. In reflexology, the foot is seen as being divided into ten zones (see illustration), which are broken down into specific reflexes or reflex points. To stimulate the zones and points, practitioners walk, rotate, roll, pivot, and flex the fingers and thumbs, applying pressure to the problem area. These techniques can improve circulation and promote healing throughout the body.

Reflexology can bring about deep relaxation. It may be particularly helpful with symptoms of premenstrual syndrome (PMS), according to studies. It's said to also help detoxify the body. A visit to the re-

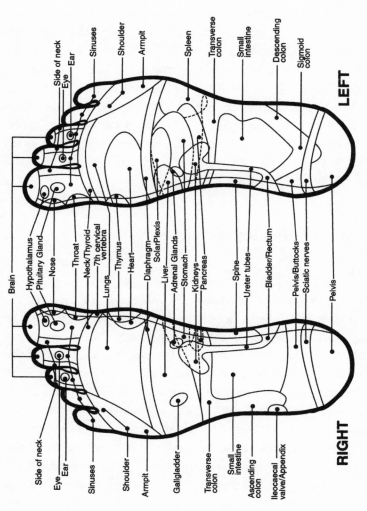

Reflexology Map

In reflexology, pressure is applied to reflex points on the soles (shown), tops and sides of the feet, as well as the hands and ears, to stimulate healing in corresponding energy zones, organs and organ systems. (Source: *Encyclopedia of Healing Therapies* by Anne Woodham and Dr. David Peters. Dorling Kindersley)

Labels on the left foot (LEFT): Side of neck, Eye, Ear, Sinuses, Shoulder, Armpit, Spleen, Transverse colon, Small intestine, Descending colon, Sigmoid colon, Brain, Hypothalamus, Pituitary Gland, Nose, Throat, Neck/Thyroid, 7th cervical vertebra, Lungs, Thymus, Heart, Diaphragm, SolarPlexis, Liver, Adrenal Glands, Stomach, Kidneys, Pancreas, Spine, Ureter tubes, Bladder/Rectum, Pelvis/Buttocks, Sciatic nerves, Pelvis

Labels on the right foot (RIGHT): Side of neck, Eye, Ear, Sinuses, Shoulder, Armpit, Gallgladder, Transverse colon, Small intestine, Ascending colon, Ileocaecal valve/Appendix flexologist will last anywhere from a half hour to an hour. You may be sitting in a chair or lying down while the practitioner examines and works on your feet and hands. Olatunde begins by administering paraffin therapy to first relax muscles in the hands and feet in order to reach nerves more readily. With a client lying on a reclining chair, she applies pressure to reflex points that correspond to systems throughout the body. If she feels "stress" or blockage in any area, she will return to that point. Olatunde recommends at least one session a week for five sessions, then a session every other week or once a month for preventive maintenance. She has helped clients alleviate high blood pressure and she believes reflexology can serve as an effective complement to conventional cancer treatment. "The body cannot heal itself unless it's in a state of rest and relaxation," she notes. Reflexology gets you there.

Healing with Energy

Acupuncture

A major component of Traditional Chinese Medicine (TCM), acupuncture uses specialized needles, placed in specific points, to free blockages in the energy system of the body. When energy is freely flowing along the twelve energy pathways, or meridians, of the body, our systems are in balance. When energy is blocked, our organs and essence, or substances, may not receive the qi *(chi)* or life force that sustains them, and this can cause disease. Over five thousand years ago, Chinese healers began to identify pressure points that, when stimulated, had a healing effect on other parts of the body. In the process, they discovered a complex system of meridians, organs, and essences (see illustration) which relate to each other in a balanced, harmonious network. The acupuncture needle, in essence, allows the practitioner to participate in this system, stimulating our chi, relieving blockages, and restoring the body to yin-yang balance and self-healing.

Acupuncture, which means "to prick a needle," has been observed

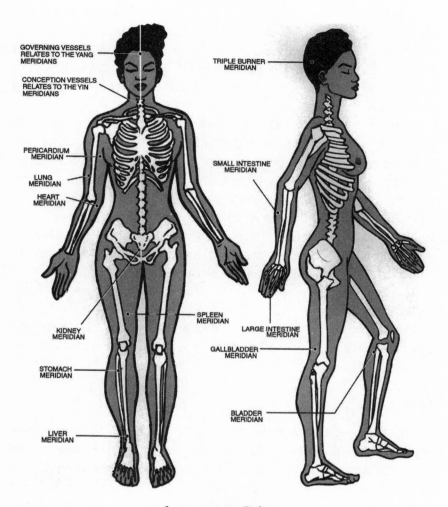

Acupuncture Points

Acupuncturists insert acupuncture needles in specific points along 14 major meridians, or energy pathways, of the body in order to stimulate the flow of *qi* (chi) or life force. This technique restores balance and healing.

(Source: *Encyclopedia of Healing Therapies* by Anne Woodham and Dr. David Peters. Dorling Kindersley)

to effectively relieve pain and nausea associated with surgery. It can also help with arthritis, asthma, many "female" problems, headaches, addictions, and plain ole stress. As a complement to conventional cancer treatment, acupuncture may be very useful. Among other benefits, acupuncture stimulates the release of endorphins, natural pain killers, and the immune system.

During a visit to the acupuncturist's office, the practitioner will not just focus on the symptom at hand, but read six pulses felt in the arm and examine your tongue to evaluate the health of your meridian system. Treatment may include the placement of burning herbs on acupuncture points, known as moxibustion, or electro-acupuncture. Besides a slight tingle or discomfort, acupuncture needles do not cause pain. One session may last an hour; treatment may last for weeks or months. Side effects, which are usually short-lived, may include dizziness, weakness or an increase in your symptoms.

Acupuncture may be practiced by several different types of healers including doctors of Oriental medicine (OMDs), naturopaths, osteopaths, and medical doctors trained in the practice. Be sure your practitioner is licensed and explains the number of treatments required.

Acupressure

This Chinese massage therapy also aims to restore energy flow and balance to the body by stimulating specific pressure points along the meridian system. However, practitioners mainly use the thumbs, fingers, and knuckles to apply pressure to the points that are the keys to healing. Acupressurists pinch, press, rub, roll, and stretch the skin and muscles in order to stimulate pressure points and trigger points that correspond to various organs and systems throughout the body. Within seconds or minutes, this pressure eases tension, encouraging blood and chi flow. Acupressure can ease aches and pains of all kinds, relieve nausea, and boost well-being.

At-Home Acupressure

Before you reach into your medicine cabinet, consider trying simple acupressure exercises to relieve painful discomfort at home. There is no special equipment required. All you need is a relaxing space and comfortable clothing. It is also best if nails are trimmed to avoid scratching or bruising yourself.

For each step, apply pressure for one to three minutes. To relieve cramps, bloating, or fluid retention

- Sit up and prop your back against a chair, or lie down on your back and rest legs on a chair.
- Place your left hand in the crease of the groin where your hip joins your thigh, about halfway between the hipbone and the outside edge of the pubic bone. Your left hand remains here for each step. Gently press and hold your right hand into the spot just above the knee on the connecting leg.
- Press and hold your right hand into a spot just below the inner part of your knee.
- Keeping your left hand in the crease of the groin, take your right hand and hold the inside of your shin (about four finger widths above the ankle).
- Move your right hand down to your foot and press your fingers into the edge of your instep. To find the point, follow the big toe bone down until you hit a small, prominent bone.
- Hold your big toe (front and back) over the nail with your right hand.

(Source: *hhtp://www.healthy.net/library/books/lark/ acu_crmp.htm*)

Laying On of hands

In this technique, a healer uses her or his hands as a channel for healing energy. By passing the hands over a person's body and touching it in strategic spots, the healer can help the individual tap into universal energy in order to stablize their own. The flow of energy helps to correct imbalances or blockages of energy that underlie illness of a spiritual, mental, emotional, or physical nature. Our energy fields are, of course, invisible to most of us. However, energetic healers are able to detect imbalances by noting irregularities in skin temperature or muscle tightness, for example. Some psychic healers may actually see the fields, also referred to as auras, which they can use to diagnose physical and emotional problems.

Healing with Chakras

Ever wonder why you sometimes become physically sick during an emotional crisis? Your thoughts and feelings control the energy flow within and around you. Chakras (a word derived from the ancient Hindu language Sanskrit meaning "wheel of light") are energy centers located deep within the center of your body. There are seven major chakras. Each one is linked to a particular part of the body and is influenced by specific thoughts and feelings. There is a chakra for each "issue" that you commonly think about, from your finances and career to your lifestyle and relationships. There is a specific color for each energy center. Ancient yogis would wear a stone of a specific color to influence the energy of a particular chakra. Below is a brief overview of the seven major chakras. You may be surprised to find that that stressful "issue" you've been struggling with is associated with the same part of the body that's been achy recently. If so, try focusing on the related chakra during meditation or prayer. Become more conscious of your thoughts, keeping in mind the critical role they play in your overall health.

The Root Chakra. Located at the base of your spine, your root chakra is related to issues of physical security and is affected by your thoughts and feelings about finances, career, home, physical safety, basic necessities, and personal possessions. The color of this chakra is a brilliant ruby red. It treats inertia.

The Sacral Chakra. The second major chakra is found midway between your navel and the base of your spine. The color of the sacral chakra is orange. Your thoughts and feelings in regard to physical desires, addictions, physical health, and appearance affect the sacral chakra. It heals depression.

The Solar Plexus Chakra. The third major chakra is found right behind the navel. The color of this chakra is bright yellow. Your thoughts and feelings about power and control affect your solar plexus chakra. It treats unresolved feelings.

The Heart Chakra. The fourth chakra, located in the center of the chest, is a beautiful shade of green. Thoughts and feelings concerning relationships, love, people attachments (codependency), and the willingness to forgive, affect the heart chakra. It heals nervousness.

The Throat Chakra. The fifth major chakra is in the Adam's apple area and is sky blue in color. The throat chakra is affected by thoughts and feelings related to being honest with yourself and others, your artistic abilities, speaking your mind, and asking for your needs to be met (by God, friends, coworkers, yourself). It treats insomnia or overactivity.

The Brow Chakras. The sixth is also known as the "third eye." The color of this chakra is indigo. It relates to perception, intuition, dignity, self-respect, and tolerance. It heals addictions.

The Crown Chakra. Located at the top of the head, the crown chakra relates to spiritual development, commitment, and idealism. It's color is violet. It deals with compulsive behavior.

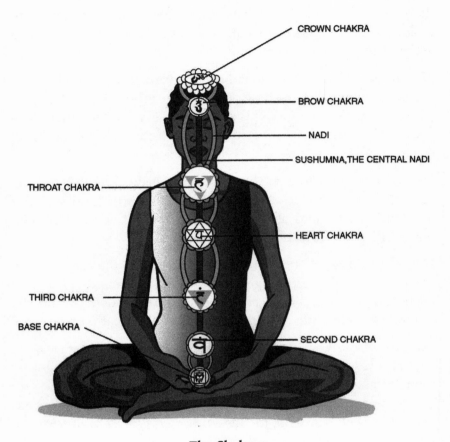

CROWN CHAKRA

BROW CHAKRA

NADI

SUSHUMNA, THE CENTRAL NADI

THROAT CHAKRA

HEART CHAKRA

THIRD CHAKRA

BASE CHAKRA

SECOND CHAKRA

The Chakras

According to some schools of Yoga, seven chakras, or energy centers, ascend along the center of the body from the groin to the top of the head. Concentrating on these chakras during yoga or meditation stimulates the flow of energy and healing. (Source: *Encyclopedia of Healing Therapies* by Anne Woodham and Dr. David Peters. Dorling Kindersley)

Wading in the Waters: Hydrotherapy

Ever used a steam room, taken an Epsom salt bath, or applied a cold or hot compress? Then you've benefited from one of the most versatile forms of natural healing: hydrotherapy. Basically, hydrotherapy means using water, in any form, to heal. The Egyptians frequently indulged in healing waters for rejuvenation. Today, spas commonly offer special body wraps and steam baths. The benefits of H_2O are legion. Warm water or steam can increase circulation, relax muscles, and generally soothe the body. Cold water relieves pain and swelling. Externally, water stimulates; internally, it purifies. You can apply hydrotherapy at home by yourself or in a spa setting with the help of a hydrotherapist.

Though water can be enormously comforting, you should avoid hot and cold extremes if you have diabetes, hypertension, heart disease, or if you are pregnant. Common forms of hydrotherapy include:

Baths and Whirlpools. Few things feel better at the end of the day than a good soak in the tub. To further the healing benefit, you can add aromatic oils to soothe or stimulate, or mineral salts such as Epsom for purification. You can also take a quick cool dip to alleviate pain or fatigue. At a spa, you can also enjoy the pulsating jet of a Jacuzzi or try thalassotherapy, a bath that utilizes seaweed for deep cleansing. Baths are especially good for arthritis and other forms of muscle or joint pain.

Showers. Hot or cold showers can invigorate the body and relieve pain. Alternating between hot and cold temperatures is another way to rejuvenate and take advantage of the body's response to the changing temperatures.

Steam. Steam rooms or baths promote sweating and, according to natural healers, the elimination of wastes and toxins through the skin.

Body Wraps. This form of hydrotherapy consists of wrapping the body from neck to toe in towels that are soaked in a solution of warm water and any combination of herbs and minerals. Wrapped in shrouds, you rest for up to an hour, allowing the warmth to relax your body and the herbs to be absorbed. This process is designed to promote the release of toxins.

Ice/Heat Packs. You can use a hot compress to soothe a sore muscle or relieve menstrual cramps. Cold compresses or ice packs are useful to relieve a fever or minimize swelling.

Colonic Irrigation Therapy. Also known as colon cleansing or simply, colonics, colonic irrigation therapy uses water to cleanse the colon of waste. Colonic therapists believe that stagnant waste can accumulate and harm the body if toxins are absorbed from the colon into the bloodstream. To eliminate the waste, therapists use a machine to flush the colon with water or a solution of water and herbs; the water and waste then drain out. You can also administer colonic enemas at home. To benefit from colon therapy, you may need to do a series of colonics. However, colonics can disrupt the body's water balance and deplete the body of electrolytes, so be sure to consult an experienced practitioner who can explain the pros and cons.

Movement Therapies

Moving the body rhythmically to music helps us heal by allowing us to experience our bodies in different ways and express our emotions through movement. Dance therapists use a particular form of movement, often in conjunction with physical therapy or psychotherapy, to help children, adults, and elderly with physical or emotional challenges. However, some "healing dances" have more spiritual roots that hark back to African traditions.

Resources

American Academy of Medical Acupuncture, 5820 Wilshire Boulevard, Suite 500, Los Angeles, CA 90036; (800) 521-2262.

The American Academy of Osteopathy, 3500 DePauw Boulevard, Suite 1080, Indianapolis, IN 46268-1136.

American Chiropractic Association, 1701 Clarendon Boulevard, Arlington, VA 22209.

American Massage Therapy Association, 820 Davis Street, Suite 100, Evanston, IL, 60201.

American Osteopathic Association, 142 East Ontario Street, Chicago, IL 60611, (800) 621-1773.

International Chiropractors Association, 1110 North Glebe Road, Suite 1000, Arlington, VA 22201.

International Institute of Reflexology, 5650 First Avenue North, PO Box 12642, St. Petersburg, FL 33733-2642.

National Acupuncture and Oriental Medicine Alliance, 14637 Starr Road, SE, Olalla, WA 98359.

National Certification Board for Therapeutic Massage and Bodywork, 8201 Greenboro Drive, Suite 300, McLean, VA 22102.

National College of Naturopathic Medicine, 11231 SE Market Street, Portland, OR 97216.

Reflexology Research, PO Box 35820, Albuquerque, NM 87176-5820.

The Encyclopedia of Bodywork: From Acupressure to Zone Therapy, by Elaine Stillerman, LMT (Checkmark Books).

Chapter 7

~

Your Periods and PMS

NATURAL WOMAN: MAXINE CAMPBELL (TEHUTI)

Beginning in her late teens, Maxine Campbell always had problem periods. With a week of bloating and headaches before her menses, bleeding that lasted eight "long, hemorrhaging days," and a week to recover, Maxine was left with only one normal week per month. Severe cramps and bleeding forced her to routinely stay home a couple of days from school, and later, from work. Over-the-counter painkillers barely alleviated her symptoms, which also included nausea and water retention. "It was just unbearable," she recalls. Unbearable lasted for seventeen years.

Like many black women, Maxine had long been eating meat. She also says that at the time she had a "bad attitude." In 1992 a friend who noticed her mood swings turned her on to a holistic health consultant, Queen Afua of Brooklyn, New York. The friend faxed her materials about various pelvic conditions—fibroids, cysts— and the benefits of a natural lifestyle, which motivated Maxine to make a change. She did not want to have a hysterectomy like her mother had had. So she followed Afua's twenty-one-day natural liv-

129

ing fast consisting of fresh fruit and vegetable juice to start, then made more permanent changes in her diet. Maxine eliminated all animal products and limited her intake of refined starches. Within four months, she noticed a difference. "My menses went from eight to three days," she explains. "No bloating. No water retention. No mood swings or bad attitude."

Maxine—who now goes by the Khemetic (Egyptian) name Te-huti—continues to fast, just eating vegetables, fruit, salads, and juice, for three days before each period, and she administers her own enema to cleanse during one of those three days. In addition to the natural eating habits, she walks and does African dance for exercise, and she meditates daily. Meditation gave her the clarity and focus to realize that since childhood, she had long been in the dark about her body and reproductive functions. Maxine's mother, a reverend, did not talk to her about such matters, leaving Maxine's many questions about womanhood unanswered. "Sex was not discussed," she says. "So I didn't feel comfortable about that topic. It was a suppressed emotion."

Through positive affirmation, meditation, and visualization, Maxine has deepened her healing. She visualizes herself feeling light and comfortable during her periods. "When you know that [your period is] getting ready to come you go through the 'oh god here it comes. This is not going to be all right. I'm gonna have hurt,'" she notes. "And before you know it you've set yourself up for the whole process. So I wanted to reverse that process and make it more positive."

Maxine's holistic approach has given her more physical energy and a positive outlook. "When you become conscious and aware you become responsible, and you become your own reliable source for healing," she says.

Our Cycles, Ourselves

Like the moon phases, the rising and setting of the sun, and the seasons, our bodies function in cycles. Beginning with our first periods, our little girls' bodies begin to take on a woman's rhythm that is in harmony with nature. Each month, our brains tell our pituitary glands to release hormones, setting off a chain of events that prepares our wombs for making a baby. If the opportunity for conception and implantation passes, the body returns to its equilibrium until the next month.

For many sisters, however, this miracle of nature is accompanied by all sorts of "female problems"—pain, excessive bleeding, cramping, moodiness. Though the changes our bodies go through are natural—even sacred—they may also reveal underlying problems or imbalances in the mind-body system. Our monthly symptoms may be more than mere female problems to endure or suppress but messages that we need to take better care of ourselves physically, emotionally, and spiritually. When we listen to the messages, our womanhood need not be fraught with discomfort and dis-ease but rather with a renewed sense of our power and creativity.

Natural Healing Is Our History

Native cultures throughout the world celebrate the arrival of a woman's first period and honor menstruating females as sacred and wise. Indigenous Africans liken the womb and its functions to the Earth, our respected mother and home, says Sobonfu Somé in her book about African traditions, *Welcoming Spirit Home*. In fact, in the Dagara tribe of West Africa, Somé explains, community members perform a symbolic cleansing ritual to protect the wombs of women who plan to have children from negative energy.

However, because of myths as old as Eve, many of us were raised to dread our periods and feel ashamed about our womanhood. African-American women tend to have more negative than positive feelings about menstruation. Studies comparing the attitudes of black and white girls toward their periods reveal that young black females are more likely to associate shame and uncleanliness with their menstrual flow. Women "on the rag" still believe themselves to be "dirty" or "unclean" and they may be treated that way by others.

Perhaps this is one reason why black women are more likely to use douches than white women, despite the fact that douching is not necessary for health and may be detrimental to it (see "Dangers of Douching"). Shaped by patriarchal myths, our negative cultural beliefs toward menstruation greatly influence our experience of this natural reproductive event.

Self-Awareness Tool

The Day You Got Your Period

One 29-year-old sister recalls that on the day she first got her period at age 10, her mother's immediate reaction was to say, "I'm sorry." How was the arrival of your menstrual period received? What words/feelings do you associate with it? Take a few minutes to think about and write down your response:

_____

_____

_____

_____

_____

In spite of the many negative ideas many sisters have been taught to associate with menstruation, there's evidence that some black women do retain positive notions about it. In *Walkin' Over Medicine*, anthropologist Loudell Snow states that traditionally, many black women tend to view the menstrual period in the following ways: as a barometer of overall well-being, as cleansing and necessary for health maintenance, and as "natural" and in harmony with nature's rhythms. These more positive ideas are ones to keep in mind as we learn more about the miracle of our reproductive cycles and how to heal them when they are not functioning well.

Case in point: When Gwendolyn Goldsby Grant, EdD, began menstruating as a young girl, her family threw her a party. "Everybody gave me gifts and congratulated me because I had started my period and stepped up on a new stage of my life," recalls the psychologist, certified sex counselor, and columnist for *Essence*. Because of the education and support she received from her mother regarding her sexuality, Dr. Grant was able to embrace her period as part of her power as a woman. "My period represented a time when I became in charge of the real *femaleness* of my body," Grant explains. "Every time I got my period, I felt more and more like I was a woman in charge of my body." Instead of calling it a curse, Grant considered her period a friend.

Menstruation

The beginning of our periods marks the first day of the menstrual cycle. At this time, declining levels of the reproductive hormones estrogen and progesterone cause the thickened lining of the uterus, called the endometrium, to shed and leave the body through the vagina. The sloughing of endometrial blood and tissue, aided by uterine contractions, takes anywhere from 2 to 8 days. From the first day of your cycle, even as you menstruate, another egg develops in the ovaries. Ovulation occurs at midcycle, most often on day 14, when the egg passes into the fallopian tubes and begins making its way into the uterus. Over the next 2 weeks, in response to increasing hormone levels, the endometrium thickens. By the twenty-eighth day or so, one of two things happen: A fertilized egg attaches itself to the endometrium, where it will grow, or the unfertilized egg leaves the body, followed by the blood and tissue known as your period.

Before your period, you may experience breast tenderness and bloating as your body retains fluid to prepare for a developing fetus. Many women—some estimate the majority of women—also notice stomach cramping, anxiety, sadness, and fatigue among other changes during this time. Some people with asthma, bad pain, arthritis and lupus, have intensified symptoms. Once the period begins, you may experience more cramping and a heavy blood loss that leads to fatigue. For some, these hormonally driven changes are not too bothersome; for others, they wreak havoc! If your cycle does not appear to be regular or if period-related symptoms concern you, you can learn and adopt natural ways to correct or alleviate them. Your period is not separate from any other part of you, so as you consider its flow, you should also be aware of how your diet, lifestyle, stress level, and emotions may be affecting it.

Common Cycle-Related Concerns

PMS

Premenstrual syndrome, or PMS, is the name given to the hormone-related physical and emotional changes that women experience cyclically—about a week before the menstrual period begins each month. No one knows for sure why PMS affects some women and not others. Though medical experts long attributed PMS to being in women's heads, researchers have recently learned a few things about potential causes. One is that women who complain of PMS may have lower levels of the brain chemical serotonin—which affects mood—during the premenstrual phase of the cycle than women who don't. Another theory points to an unusual response to the shifts in the hormones estrogen and progesterone during PMS. The problem most often affects women in their twenties and thirties and may get worse over time. A small percentage of women have a severe form of PMS, premenstrual dysphoric disorder, that interferes with normal functioning. Most, however, experience some combination of the following symptoms:

Abdominal bloating	Fluid retention
Acne	Food cravings (sugar, salt)
Anxiety	Headache/migraine
Breast swelling/pain	Insomnia
Clumsiness	Irritability

Constipation	Lethargy
Depression	Nausea/vomiting
Diarrhea	Rage/anger
Difficulty concentrating	Sexual arousal
Fatigue	Weight gain

Some holistic healers believe that because the womb is our center of creativity—where we literally "create" life—stifling of our creativity can trigger physical symptoms in the uterus, such as fibroids (see Chapter 8). Others, including the holistic obstetrician-gynecologist Christiane Northrup, feel that our menstrual cycles are connected to the cycling and processing of our emotions. Perhaps that is why women feel more "emotional" during the PMS period. Resistance to facing and dealing with all of our emotions may be the underlying cause of cycle-related health problems. Though we may be tempted to dismiss our mood swings as "just PMS," those feelings may be the very ones we need to pay more attention to. The intensity of our feelings during this time may be uncomfortable or even frightening. But think of it this way: PMS may simply be the body's way of getting our attention, urging us to take care of unfinished or unhealed emotional business.

Experts note that black women tend to have more of the emotional symptoms associated with PMS, such as irritability and moodiness, than white women. Our choices in natural remedies should emphasize emotional healing.

Natural Prevention and Treatment
• *Lifestyle/Stress Management.* Get some exercise most days of the week to stave off depression and lift your mood. Do the exercise outside so you can to take in the healing light of the sun, which can trigger positive changes in your brain chemistry. Get the sleep you need and explain to your mate and children that you may need more TFM (time for me) than usual.

• *Nutrition.* Avoid sugar, salt, caffeine, and alcohol, which can exacerbate PMS symptoms. Plan balanced meals including minimally processed complex carbohydrates (found in whole grains and vegetables), protein, and minimal fat. If you eat dairy products, stop eating them for three months to see if you experience relief, or switch to organic dairy foods.

• *Supplements/Herbs.* Take a multivitamin-mineral supplement that contains magnesium and vitamin B_6. Extra calcium may also help. Women in a St. Luke's-Roosevelt Hospital Center study published in 1998 reported significant relief from PMS symptoms after taking calcium carbonate supplements for three months. Try essential fatty acids in the form of fish oil or flaxseed oil supplements. Evening primrose oil is another essential fatty acid that works for a lot women. Talk to your ob-gyn or other licensed health care provider to determine if you might benefit from natural progesterone (not to be confused with synthetic progestin) in capsule or cream form.

• *Mind-Body.* Practice the relaxation technique that works best for you (e.g., deep breathing, meditation, progressive muscle relaxation, see pages 96–97) for at least 10 minutes every day. One study published in the *Journal of Obstetrician-Gynecologists and Neonatal Nurses* in 1999 showed that by joining a support group and getting educated about their menstrual cycles, women reduced their PMS symptoms. Another study demonstrated that three months of cognitive behavioral therapy—a form of talk therapy—helped women eliminate emotional and physical symptoms of PMS.

• *Hands-On Healing.* Practitioners of reflexology, acupuncture, acupressure, and chiropractic have helped women alleviate PMS.

Cramps (Dysmenorrhea)

Most women experience some pain in the lower abdomen just before and/or during menstruation. This pain or cramping is known as dysmenorrhea (meaning "painful flow") and it comes in two forms. Primary dysmenorrhea is the term used to describe painful uterine contractions that occur during menstruation; secondary dysmenorrhea is abdominal pain that is associated with some other pelvic problem or disease such as endometriosis (see Chapter 8). Research suggests that women with primary dysmenorrhea may have higher levels of prostaglandins, the naturally occurring fatty acids that stimulate uterine contractions during our periods. As if the cramping wasn't bad enough, some sisters also experience nausea, headache, and dizziness.

Natural Prevention and Treatment

• *Lifestyle/Stress Management.* Exercise most days of the week to relax muscles, improve circulation, and keep stress to a minimum. Also get plenty of rest.

• *Nutrition.* In studies, women who consumed fish oils had reduced cramps so try adding fatty-acid-rich cold-water fish like salmon and swordfish to your diet. Avoid high-fat foods (meat, dairy) and those containing partially hydrogenated oils (such as margarine).

• *Supplements/Herbs.* In addition to a multivitamin-mineral supplement, extra vitamins B_6, E, C, and calcium, and magnesium may help during your period. Various herbs (e.g., dong quai) may relieve cramps; consult a licensed practitioner about combinations and dosages.

• *Mind-Body.* Practicing yoga may help relieve cramps by relieving muscle tension and fluid congestion in the pelvic area.

• *Hands-On Healing.* Those hot-water bottles or heating pads your mother recommended often work. Acupuncture treatments may also be useful for severe cramps.

Heavy periods (Menorrhagia)

If you bleed excessively, going through several tampons or pads—and sometimes your clothes—in one hour, you may have a hormone imbalance or underlying pelvic illness such as fibroids or endometriosis (see Chapter 8). Having an IUD may also trigger heavy, prolonged periods.

• *Lifestyle.* Exercise to reduce body fat and circulating estrogens. Weight-training twice per week can help you build muscle and cut fat (you may want to work around the severest period days).

• *Nutrition.* Eat more fiber-rich carbohydrates found in vegetables, fruits, and beans. Cut down on processed foods including refined carbohydrates or "starches" (most bread, pasta), which may disturb your hormonal balance. If you eat meat or dairy, stop eating them for a few months to see if symptoms lessen.

• *Supplements.* Take a multivitamin-mineral formula, plus vitamins A, C, and E. Consider natural progesterone, according to your practitioner's instructions.

• *Hands-On Healing.* Try acupuncture.

No Periods (Amenorrhea)

Most teenage girls begin their periods by age 16, if not long before (these days some sisters begin menstruating as early as age 8!). Until that time we have what's known as primary amenorrhea and it is quite normal. At first, our periods can stop and start irregularly as our bodies grow and mature. If, however, our periods do not begin by age 16, they may be delayed by some hormonal imbalance or other physical problem that a health care provider must diagnose.

When our periods cease for months at a time in adulthood, we have what's called secondary amenorrhea. The most obvious reason for skipped periods is pregnancy. After age 35 or 40, our periods may also become irregular because of perimenopause, or the stage before menopause (see Chapter 10). Other causes include rapid weight gain or loss, vigorous athletic training, use of oral contraceptives, extreme stress, or a medical condition (ovarian cysts, diabetes). At times, skipped periods are simply unexplained. If your periods pause for no apparent reason, you should see a health care provider. Dr. Northrup believes that amenorrhea could stem from negative feelings about becoming a woman.

• *Lifestyle.* If you exercise every day, cut back to every other day to see if your period returns. If you have recently gained or lost a lot of weight, talk to a nutritionist or other provider about how your weight change might be affecting your health—and how you can eat and exercise more moderately.

• *Nutrition.* Eat a balanced diet including natural sources of iron (beans, soy, sea vegetables) to prevent anemia, a potential cause of amenorrhea. If you have Type 2 diabetes, talk to your provider about nutritional changes you can make to stabilize your blood sugar and your health. Natural progesterone may also help; talk to your provider.

• *Supplements/Herbs.* If you are anemic, talk to your provider about taking iron supplements in addition to a multivitamin-mineral supplement. Iron supplements should be taken only temporarily to correct anemia.

• *Mind-Body Methods.* Stay in control of stress through deep breathing, meditation, or progressive muscle relaxation. If stress feels overwhelming, talk to a therapist. Celebrate your womanhood by creating or joining a sister circle, and reading about the achievements of black women in books such as *I Dream a World*.

• *Hands-On Healing.* Acupuncture may unblock any stagnation in your *qi* or life force that could cause amenorrhea.

The Womb and Pelvis

The word "womb" evokes images of nurturance, protection, comfort, and motherhood. Our wombs are powerful centers, where the miracle of life occurs. In the indigenous West African tradition, according to Sobonfu Somé, the womb is considered the home of a new spirit entering the world. To prepare the home, many traditional African women make the effort to correct any negative feelings they might have about their femininity in order to safeguard the womb. The community also honors the womb through rituals and prayer.

Yet this vital organ has become the most disposable one in hospitals across the United States where hysterectomy is the second most common surgery after C-sections. Black women are more likely to undergo this major surgical procedure than white women. The most common reason for hysterectomy is fibroid tumors, but removal of the womb may also result from other reproductive disorders. The high rate of hysterectomy speaks to not only the disdain many medical doctors have for an organ that is seen as having one function—making babies—but also to the quick-fix mentality of such doctors who don't fully understand or appreciate the female body. Medical science has few answers for common pelvic problems—fibroids, endometriosis, ovarian cysts—and there are many questions.

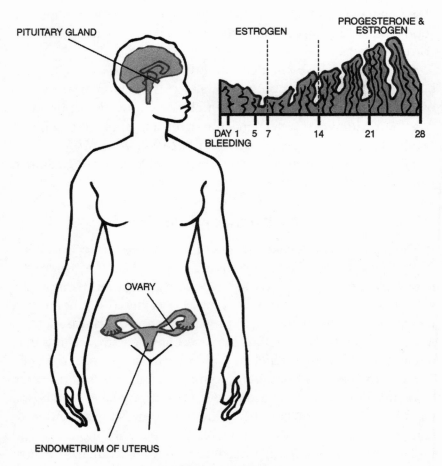

The Menstrual Cycle

The pituitary gland in the brain secretes hormones that increase estrogen levels during the menstrual cycle. Midway through the cycle, the ovaries release an egg that is either fertilized and implanted in the uterus or released from the body with menstrual flow.

Our uterus and ovaries are important beyond their reproductive functions. They produce hormones throughout our lives, even after menopause. These creative organs have energy and purpose beyond their medically defined functions. Natural healers consider the effects of an unnatural diet and unnatural suppression of emotion and creativity on the pelvic organs. Strategies for healing must return to the source.

Common Womb Concerns

Endometriosis

Endometriosis is a baffling condition in which cells that normally line the uterine wall (endometrium) grow outside of the uterus. These lost cells most often find a home elsewhere in the pelvis—on the ovaries, fallopian tubes, vagina, bladder, or bowel—but they can also travel to other areas of the body including the lungs and brain in rare cases. Outside the uterus, these cells do what they would do otherwise, thickening and bleeding once a month in response to hormonal changes. This activity can cause abnormal bleeding, pain, inflammation, cysts, the buildup of scar tissue, and organ damage. Endometriosis may contribute to infertility.

Many medical experts believe endometriosis is the result of retrograde menstruation—or menstruation that flows backward up through the fallopian tubes and into the pelvic cavity. Others believe it is an autoimmune response, in which the body produces antibodies against itself for no apparent reason. Still others think it is triggered by environmental toxins that act like hormones. What is known is that endometriosis appears to run in families. Some women have signs of endometriosis and no symptoms while others suffer extreme pain.

• *Lifestyle.* Exercise regularly. Take the time to examine and minimize the sources of stress in your life. Establish regular waking and sleeping patterns that coincide with nature.

• *Nutrition.* Remove meat and dairy from your diet for at least three months to note any difference in symptoms. Eat plenty of fiber-rich foods such as vegetables and whole grains; fatty-acid rich fish like salmon; and soy.

• *Supplements/Herbs.* Take a multivitamin-mineral supplement.

• *Hands-On Healing.* Acupuncture or massage may relieve pelvic pain.

Ovarian Cysts

Cysts—or small, usually fluid-filled sacs—within our ovaries are usually benign growths responding to ovulation and are quite common. This type of ovarian cyst sometimes causes pain or bleeding but typically goes away on its own within three or four months. Others are more solid, made up of blood and cells. These larger, more persistent cysts can cause extreme pain and bleeding. In rare instances cysts contain precancerous or cancerous cells that can lead to ovarian cancer.

Another ovarian condition is known as polycystic ovarian syndrome (POS). In POS, a woman's body produces an abnormally high level of male hormones or androgens, which prevents egg production and ovulation. When this occurs, cysts that would normally develop and disappear cyclically remain in the ovary, enlarging it. Symptoms include irregular or absent periods and excess facial hair growth. The cause of POS is unknown, but because many women with POS are overweight, excess body fat may be a contributing factor. Some natural healers contend that the ovaries represent our creative impulses. Healing should include the free expression of our creative instincts.

If your sister, mother, aunt, or cousin has or had ovarian cancer, you may be at increased risk for developing this malignancy. Ovarian cancer can grow quite rapidly and be symptomless until the late stages of the disease. If you notice pelvic problems of any kind, even chronic indigestion, get a checkup and work with your provider to minimize your risk. If you develop ovarian cancer, natural therapies can complement medical treatment.

• *Lifestyle.* Exercise most days of the week to reduce excess body fat, and to keep hormone levels balanced. Establish regular waking and sleeping patterns that coincide with nature. Do not use talcum powder, which has been linked to ovarian cancer.

• *Nutrition.* Avoid dairy and meat. Eat a balanced diet rich in natural foods including fresh vegetables, fruit, minimally processed whole grains, soy, nuts, and beans.

• *Supplements/Herbs.* Take a multivitamin-mineral supplement. Consider natural progesterone, according to health provider instructions.

• *Mind-Body Methods.* Meditation and journaling may help you quiet the mind in order to get back in touch with long lost creative desires that you can incorporate into daily life.

Cervical Changes

The lowermost part of the uterus, the cervix, connects the womb to the vagina. It has a small opening, covered with mucus, that protects the womb from bacteria. The cervical opening, or os, opens to let sperm in but closes as soon as an egg is fertilized. The main function of our annual Pap smear is to check the health of cervical cells. Experts refer to abnormal changes in cervical cells as dysplasia, which simply means "abnormal development" of cells or organs. Most of the time, these changes are mild and go away on their own. Less commonly, dysplasia may persist and lead to cancer.

A common but little-known infection that affects the cervix is the human papillomavirus or HPV. This virus, which is passed through skin contact, causes vaginal warts and may contribute to abnormal changes in cervical cells. In most people, the presence of HPV does not necessarily cause illness. When it does, an infection may not produce noticeable symptoms—warts, irritation—for years. However, particularly virulent strains of HPV may contribute to cell changes that lead to cervical cancer. Your physician can detect the virus through Pap smear or colposcopy (examination of the cervix using a magnifying glass and sometimes including a biopsy). Though warts can be removed by your GYN, HPV is not curable.

Black women must be particularly vigilant about getting Pap smears because we are more likely than white women to die of cervical cancers that are detected late. Cervical cancer may not show signs until it has progressed. Those signs include pelvic pain, bleeding after intercourse or between periods, and unusual discharge.

Holistic gynecologists contend that cervical problems are exacerbated—if not caused—by stress and other emotional issues, particularly relationship issues. Taking care of ourselves emotionally, spiritually, and nutritionally will help the body fight the causes of dysplasia and heal before they turn into cancer.

• *Lifestyle.* To keep your immune system strong, take the time to examine and minimize the sources of stress in your life, particularly in the area of relationships. Be sure to avoid cigarettes and secondhand smoke, as smoking raises the risk of cervical abnormalities.

• *Nutrition.* Eat a balanced diet rich in natural foods including fresh vegetables and fruits that provide antioxidants (vitamins A, C, and E, folic acid, selenium) and B complex vitamins.

• *Supplements.* Take a multivitamin/mineral supplement to maintain adequate nutrient levels.

Dangers of Douching

It is supposed to make women feel "fresh" and "clean," say the advertisements. But douching—using diluted vinegar or other solutions to "wash" the vagina—is not necessary, because vaginas are self-cleansing organs. Yet women, particularly African-American women, tend to rely heavily on douching products to wash away odors after menstruation or sexual intercourse. About two-thirds of all black females douche, according to the Centers for Disease Control and Prevention. Because douching washes away the body's own protective fluids, it puts women at risk for contracting vaginal infections. In addition, douching has been linked to other health problems, such as ectopic pregnancy, pelvic inflammatory disease, and infertility. Women who are concerned about odors (unusual odors may be the sign of a serious infection) should seek the advice of a gynecologist instead of washing their vaginal health away.

Infections of the Vagina and Urinary Tract

Our outer genitals and urinary tracts are vulnerable to infections both sexually transmitted and non–sexually transmitted. These infections are extremely common but they are all preventable. It's important to take your vaginal and urinary tract health seriously: Untreated infections are not only bothersome but certain sexually transmitted diseases can cause infertility or be passed to an unborn child during delivery. So practice good health and good hygiene: Avoid wearing wet or tight clothing, and don't douche. Be consistent about safe sex. If sex is painful, use lubrication or see your GYN. Pay attention to unusual symptoms such as changes in discharge, odor, itching, burning, or pain—and seek diagnosis and treatment immediately. Though some infections must be treated medically, a natural-healing approach can improve your overall health and help prevent recurrent infections or outbreaks.

Black women appear to have higher rates of sexually transmitted infections (SITs), and we now make up the majority of women infected with HIV. These numbers may be due to lack of awareness but also lack of control in our sexual relationships. Some holistic ob/gyns believe that infection in the vaginal areas stems, in part, from conflict over our sexuality or a relationship. Giving in to sexual pressure also exposes women to more partners who may be carrying diseases. Given the persistent sexual stereotyping of black women that leaves us with little choice between being either asexual caretaker figures and lascivious sex goddesses, it's no wonder we are conflicted about our sexual behavior and roles. Do you feel victimized by anyone close to you? Do you feel comfortable and respected in the bedroom? If you don't feel in control in your intimate relationships, you may need to confront a partner or sever an unhealthy involvement and reclaim your sexual identity.

Infections (non-STIs)

Yeast Infections. Triggered by the overgrowth of a type of yeast known as *Candida albicans,* yeast infections typically cause itching, thick white discharge, and odor. Treatment usually involves an over-the-counter medication. To prevent recurrent yeast infections, eat a natural diet low in sugar and take steps to lower stress. Natural remedies include yogurt with active cultures or lactobacillus acidophilus tablets, zinc, and vitamin C.

Bacterial Vaginosis. An abundance of bacteria in the vagina causes BV. Symptoms are white or yellow discharge and a fishy odor. Antibiotics are standard treatment; natural remedies include herbal salves available in health food stores and sitz baths to soothe irritation. To prevent recurrent infections, eat a natural diet that includes yogurt if you like it, and avoid sugar and alcohol.

Urinary Tract Infections. Caused by bacteria in the urethra or bladder, UTIs such as cystitis cause symptoms including frequent trips to the bathroom, painful urination, odor, and less commonly, blood in the urine. A UTI may go away on its own; severe ones may be treated with antibiotics. Natural remedies include cranberry juice or tablets; blueberries also help. To prevent recurrent UTIs, eat a natural diet, drink water, and practice good hygiene by wiping from front to back.

Sexually Transmitted Infections (STIs)

Disease	Cause	Risk	Treatment/Remedy
Chlamydia	*Chlamydia trachomatis* bacterium	Pelvic inflammatory disease; infertility	Antibiotics
Gonorrhea	*Neisseria gonorrhoeae* bacterium	Pelvic inflammatory disease; infertility; complications to joints, heart	Antibiotics

Disease	Cause	Risk	Treatment/Remedy
Trichomonas	*Trichomonas vaginitis*	Irritation; painful urination	Antiparasitic medication
Herpes	Herpes simplex virus	Tranmission to fetus during de-livery	Acyclovir; L-lysine (amino acid) during outbreaks; garlic; zinc; vitamin C
Syphilis	*Treponema palli-dum* bacterium	Heart disease; nerve damage; brain damage	Antibiotics
Hepatitis B	Hepatitis B virus	Chronic infection; cirrhosis; liver cancer or death	No cure; high-protein or high-carbohydrate diet
HIV/AIDS	Human immuno-deficiency virus	Opportunistic in-fections; im-munodeficiency; death	No cure; combination drug therapies; nutrition

Breast Changes

When it comes to breast health, cancer tends to be the main worry for women. But finding a malignant lump is less common than some other changes in breast tissue that you should know about. To become familiar with the natural feel of your breasts so you are able to detect unnatural changes, be sure to check your breasts monthly (see Chapter 12 to learn how to do a breast self-exam). Though most lumps are benign, you should see your doctor anyway to make sure.

Cysts. Small sacs of fluid may develop in the breast and swell just before your period in response to hormonal changes. Cysts are benign and may go away on their own but they often cause tenderness and anxiety. Natural remedies include exercise to manage weight and avoid hormonal imbalance, a low-fat natural diet, and stress management.

Fibrocystic Breasts. Several cysts that feel like small, painful lumps under the skin are called fibrocystic or benign breast changes. Symptoms increase a week before your period when estrogen and

147

progesterone levels are fluctuating. Natural remedies include exercise, eating a low-fat natural diet including sources of vitamins A and E (green vegetables, beans, nuts), avoiding caffeine and chocolate, and reducing stress. If these changes don't suffice, try evening primrose oil or fish oil supplements. Castor oil packs may also help.

Fibroadenomas. More common in black women, fibroadenomas are firm, rubbery lumps or tumors. Unlike cysts and fibrocystic changes, they do not change during the menstrual cycle or cause pain. There is no known cure for these lumps; visit your physician annually to have them monitored (you may want to have it removed if the tumor is large). Use remedies described for relief of breast discomfort.

Resources

American College of Obstetricians and Gynecologists, Office of Public Information, 409 Twelfth Street, SW, Washington, DC, 20024-2188; *www.acog.org*

American Social Health Association, PO Box 13827, Research Triangle Park, NC 27709.

National Endometriosis Association, 8585, North 76th Place, Milwaukee, WI 53223; (800) 992-3636; *www.endometriosisassn.org*

National Vaginitis Association, 220 South Cook Street, Suite 201, Barrington, IL 60010.

National Women's Health Network, 514 Tenth Street, NW, Suite 400, Washington, DC 20004.

Endometriosis: A Natural Approach, by Jo Mears (Ulysses Press).

PMS Relief: Natural Approaches to Treating Symptoms, by Judy E. Marshel, MBA, RD, CD-N, and Anne Egan (Berkley).

Sacred Women: A Guide to Heal Feminine Body, Mind and Spirit, by Queen Afua (Ballantine).

Stolen Woman: Reclaiming Our Sexuality, Taking Back Our Lives, by Gail E. Wyatt (Wiley).

Women to Woman: A Leading Gynecologist Tells You All You Need to Know about Your Body and Your Health, by Yvonne S. Thornton, MD, MPH with Jo Coudert (Plume).

Women's Bodies, Women's Wisdom: Creating Physical & Emotional Health & Healing, by Dr. Christiane Northrup (Bantam).

Chapter 8

~~~~

Freedom from Fibroids

NATURAL WOMAN: LYNETTE HINDS

When Lynette Hinds first learned she had several small fibroids in her mid-thirties, they were not giving her any trouble. But later, as the registered nurse approached her forties, her menstrual bleeding increased along with the pain during that time of the month. Her fibroids had ballooned in size. "I knew they were bigger because at that time I could feel them in my stomach," she says. "I could feel the hardness in my belly." Lynette's ob-gyn suggested surgery but because the fibroids only bothered her during menstruation, she declined.

A few years later, Lynette did undergo surgery but for another more serious condition—bowel obstruction. After the second operation in one month, she felt weak. "After I came out of the hospital, I lost a lot of weight," Lynette explains. "I was feeling really beat up on, you know. I was looking for something else." She went in search of a holistic healer to renew her strength and found the Ausar Auset Society in Brooklyn. There, she worked with practitioners of alternative medicine who advised her in making lifestyle changes, healthier nutritional choices, and taking herbs. Already a vegetarian who only indulged in animal foods during holidays, Lynette swore off the unhealthy fat for good. Under the guidance of the healers at Ausar Auset, she took herbs to first cleanse then tone her system for about a month. She also learned about finding emotional balance by releasing negative feelings such as anger and fear, and focusing on joy. "Being at peace helps you to gain more insight into how to change things in your life rather than being upset or fearful," she says. "That seems to be the foundation for improving your health." She increased the peace in her life through exercise and by practicing yoga, qigong, and an African-inspired healing dance that promotes balance. The entire program of spirituality helped her ease daily stresses and better deal with life challenges.

Within two to three months, Lynette felt her energy surge and noticed one particular fibroid symptom—frequent urination—had subsided. Her appetite, which had decreased after her surgery, was back. Today, Lynette's periods are regular and her bleeding has decreased from as many as thirteen days to five to seven days per month. Her fibroids, though not completely gone, shrank significantly. She credits her healing to being more tranquil and being committed to a healthier lifestyle. "Lifestyle has a lot to do with health," she notes. "We get angry, disturbed. If something is bothering us, we're popping pills for the stomach; we get headaches, take something for the headaches. We're not sleeping." It is the pattern, she believes, that keeps many black women sick. "We get locked into a cycle of all kinds of little problems that could really be avoided if we only pay attention to what we eat, what we drink, how we function," she notes.

The Fibroid Epidemic

Fibroids, benign tumors made of fibrous and muscular tissue that typically grow in the uterus, are very common. Most black women— some two-thirds or more—have fibroids. Compared to white women, we tend to develop fibroids at a younger age, and we are more likely to have multiple fibroids and ones of large size. It is not known what causes fibroids, but the high prevalence among black women amounts to no less than an epidemic.

For some women, fibroids present no problem. But for many others, they are a constant source of discomfort and dis-ease. Though very rarely cancerous (less than 1 percent of fibroids are malignant), fibroids can cause myriad symptoms including excessive bleeding, pain, and infertility. One study published in the *Journal of Reproductive Medicine* in July 1996 found that black women are more likely than white women to be anemic and suffer pelvic pain, constipation, and stomachaches as a result of fibroids. The presence of fibroids may also add to the worries and stresses in a woman's life, further deteriorating her well-being. Fibroids are the leading cause of hysterectomy, or removal of the uterus and sometimes the ovaries as well. This common procedure—the second most common major surgery in this country after Cesarean sections—is more often performed on black women than white women. In addition to the loss of this vital organ and its functions, hysterectomies put us at risk for complications and even death.

Conventional treatments focus on removing the uterus or the fibroids themselves, or shrinking the fibroids with hormones or by cutting off their blood supply—all sophisticated techniques that don't get at the root of the problem. Because medical experts don't completely understand what causes a fibroid to grow in the first place, there has been little focus in the medical community on preventing them before they can grow or treating them naturally, although that is changing. For example, in 1997 Columbia University researchers launched an exploratory study into the effect of traditional Chinese medicine—including the use of herbs and/or acupuncture—on fibroids. The first step in either preventing or treating fibroid tumors the natural way is to learn more about them and their possible causes.

Unnatural Causes

The growing research and speculation regarding the causes of fibroids have pointed to several potential risk factors.

Heredity

Fibroids tend to run in families. In many black households most or all of the women have fibroid tumors. However, this may have more to do with inherited behaviors (diet, inactivity, psychological factors) than with genes.

Hormone Imbalance

Because fibroids tend to grow during our childbearing years while they shrink after menopause, experts believe that estrogen levels influence their growth. Other factors that increase a woman's lifetime exposure to estrogen include early menstruation (before age 12) and late childbearing (after age 30). Poor diet and excess weight (see below) also affect hormonal balance. Black women may be more susceptible to fibroids because we begin to menstruate, on average, a year earlier than white women, eat unbalanced, high-fat diets, and carry more weight. Living largely in polluted urban communities, we may also be exposed more often to environmental chemicals that mimic hormones. However, the effect of hormones on fibroids is not fully understood.

Obesity

Excess weight may contribute to fibroids because body fat, particularly fat around the abdomen, produces estrogen. The majority of black women are overweight to some degree, which may in part explain the high prevalence of fibroids, and severity of related symptoms, in our community.

Diet

A diet high in fat and processed foods may be a major factor in the creation of fibroids. Dr. Jewel Pookrum, a holistic gynecologist specializing in integrative medicine in Atlanta, believes fibroids may be the result of a poorly functioning liver. The liver, she explains, is responsible for the breakdown of fat and protein. When this organ is stressed by a high-meat diet, it cannot properly perform its other functions, including the utilization of estrogen and removal of excess estrogens from the blood. So when black women, whose ancestors did not consume meat, do so, "they are going to have higher estrogen levels just because the liver has been asked to function in an abnormal and excessive way for years prior to the manifestation of the disease," Pookrum explains.

Anecdotally, many women have been able to shrink their fibroids through nutritional change alone. Some experts suspect that the hormones given to animals to further their growth enter our bodies when we eat animal foods including dairy products and poultry. These trace hormones may disrupt the hormonal balance in women, contributing to fibroids and other reproductive health problems. Pesticide residue may also play a role. It is most likely that diet also affects the other factors—weight and hormones—associated with fibroid growth.

Psychological/Spiritual Issues

We have a tendency to think about fibroids in purely physical terms, but holistic experts speculate that women with fibroids harbor unexpressed creative desires or emotions such as anger that manifest in the uterus. The thinking is that a fibroid or fibroids represent stagnant energy that becomes a solid mass. It is not hard to imagine that, as the caretakers of those around us and the "backbones" of our race, we black women may be even more likely than others to suppress our feelings and aspirations, which may in turn generate stress and dis-ease.

"Uterine fibroid disease is a pyscho-social disorder," says Dr. Jewel Pookrum. In her own research on patients she's seen over the past fifteen years, Pookrum has discovered that women with fibroids share similar emotional and spiritual challenges, a profile she calls the "F personality." The women tend to share four characteristics: ambivalence toward motherhood; unhealed scars from romantic relationships; work they feel does not reflect their life purpose; and a lack of nurturing or self-care. This state of consciousness, Pookrum notes, manifests in the body as fibroid tumors. Black women may be more prone to this disorder because of a subconcious fear of abandonment by one's mate and separation of mother from her children instilled in our foremothers during slavery, and passed down to us today.

Self-Awareness Tool

The Sky's the Limit

Holistic healers suggest that fibroids result, at least in part, from creative blocks. To consider the influence this conflict might have in your life and on your health, take a few minutes to answer the following:

If I could have any job in the world (or one not yet created in the world), and make sufficient money doing it, I would . . .

_____

_____

_____

_____

_____

If I could create anything in the world, I would . . .

_____

_____

_____

_____

_____

You may have already found satisfying work or created something meaningful to you at this point in your life. But if you have not, think about why not, and the effect it may be having on your body. There's no better time than now to begin to seek the instruction, advice, and support you need to follow your dreams and fulfill your life purpose.

Fibroid Signs and Symptoms

Many women may not even know they have fibroids because the tumors don't always produce symptoms. If fibroids, however, grow to a large size or are numerous, they may trigger a variety of related problems that range from unpleasant to unbearable. These include:

- Excessive menstrual bleeding
- Abdominal swelling (a paunch)
- Back pain
- Fatigue from iron deficiency
- Cramps/pelvic pain
- Pain during intercourse
- Frequent urination
- Constipation
- Hemorrhoids
- Infertility
- Pregnancy complications/miscarriage

To determine whether you have fibroids, your obstetrician/gynecologist can examine the uterus manually by simply pressing down on your abdomen. To assess the size and number of fibroids, your ob/gyn can use ultrasound or a laparoscope, a thin lighted tube inserted in the abdomen through a small incision. Fibroids range greatly in size from ones that are barely perceptible to others that weigh as much as twenty-five pounds or more. Physicians typically compare them to the size of fruit or to the size of a developing fetus. It is important to see your ob-gyn annually so that she can catch fibroids before they get so large or numerous that they interfere with your health and well-being.

Fibroid Types

Tumors can grow in different areas of your uterus—inside the uterus, within the muscles of the uterine walls, or on the outside of the uterus. Experts have identified and named several fibroid types:

Submucosal. These fibroids grow inside the uterine lining or endometrium. Because of their location, they can trigger excessive menstrual bleeding.

Intramural. These fibroids grow within the uterine wall itself. Depending on their size, these fibroids may or may not cause symptoms.

Subserosal. These grow on the outer surface of the uterus and may be attached by a stalk. If these fibroids place pressure on another organ such as the rectum or bladder, they can cause symptoms like frequent urination or kidney problems.

Cervical. A minority of fibroids—about 5 percent—develop in the cervical area. This could contribute to painful intercourse.

The actual names of these fibroids don't mean as much as their locations. The placement and size of a fibroid may impinge on the bladder, causing urinary problems and even kidney disease. Submucosal fibroids may cause uterine contractions or prevent the successful implantation of a fertilized egg, raising the risk of infertility or miscarriage.

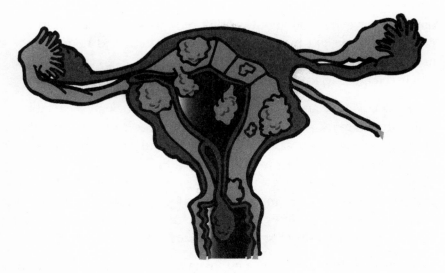

Fibroid Types

There are a few different types of fibroids, or benign tumors—ones that grow inside the uterus, outside the uterus, inside the uterine lining or endometrium, within the walls of the uterus or in the cervix. (Source: *Women's Bodies, Women's Wisdom* by Christiane Northrup, MD. Bantam)

Natural Cures

While fibroids are quite common, they are not natural. Fibroids are not necessarily life-threatening but they can be life-draining. Regardless of whether or not your fibroid or fibroids produce symptoms, the underlying cause—nutritional, hormonal, emotional, spiritual, or some combination of these—is real enough to have created an entity where one did not exist. The presence of the fibroid is expressing something you may need to pay attention to.

Natural fibroid treatment, like most natural healing strategies, is not immediate.

Lifestyle. Take the time to identify life stresses and how you can minimize them. Not only does stress contribute to any physical illness but excessive stress may make it more difficult for you to take the best care of yourself (get enough rest, eat right, etc.). Exercise most days of the week for 30 minutes or more. This will not only help you manage your weight but also increase circulation and help balance hormone levels. If you are overweight, increase exercise and make dietary changes to lose extra pounds gradually.

Nutrition. Eat balanced meals containing green leafy vegetables, fruit, whole grains, soy, beans, and peas. Dr. Pookrum recommends bitter vegetables such as endive, escarole, and turnip and mustard greens to support healthy liver and gallbladder function.

Boost essential fatty acids by eating fish (salmon, mackerel), nuts, and seeds (flaxseed). Eliminate high-fat foods (all dairy, most or all meat), sugar, salt, caffeine, and alcohol. Also, try eliminating wheat for a couple of months to see if it alleviates symptoms.

Supplements. In addition to a multivitamin-mineral supplement, B-complex vitamins, vitamins C and E, calcium, and magnesium may help ease symptoms. If you suffer fatigue, have your blood tested for iron-deficiency anemia and talk to your health care provider about taking extra iron.

Herbs. Practitioners of traditional Chinese medicine have successfully helped women shrink or eliminate their fibroids with herbal remedies. Many different herbs such as raspberry leaf may be used to cope with the underlying cause or symptoms of fibroids. Always consult a licensed herbalist for recommendations.

Mind-Body Methods. Consistently use techniques such as meditation and deep breathing to keep stress at bay. Yoga can also ease tension and boost circulation to the womb. Dr. Pookrum encourages her clients to join support groups where women can build the confidence they need to change their life work or other stressful circumstance.

Hands-On Healing. Try acupuncture or hydrotherapy.

Should I Have My Fibroid Removed?

Though women should always consider all of their options and learn about lifestyle changes that can help reduce fibroids, in some cases, symptoms may be so severe that medical intervention becomes necessary. Nonsurgical methods or surgery may be indicated if fibroids

- Cause extreme pain.
- Cause excessive bleeding, or severe bladder or pelvic pressure.
- Cause infertility.
- Turn into cancerous tumors (less than 1 percent of cases).

See your gynecologist. A simple ultrasound can determine the size and location of the fibroids, and help you and your provider decide whether a myomectomy (removal of fibroid) or new noninvasive techniques such as arterial embolization (shrinking of tumors) is your best option. Hysterectomy (removal of uterus and sometimes ovaries) should be your last resort.

Resources

The Hysterectomy Educational Resources and Services (HERS) Foundation, 422 Bryn Mawr Avenue, Bala Cynwyd, PA 19004.

The National Women's Health Network, 514 Tenth Street, NW, Suite 400 Washington, DC 20004.

Natural Treatment of Fibroid Tumors and Endometriosis, by Susan M. Lark, MD, (Keats Good Health Guide).

Chapter 9

❦

In the Family Way:
Pregnancy and Childbirth

NATURAL WOMAN: KWASAUSYA KHEPERA

When Kwasausya Khepera learned she was pregnant back in 1991, like many mothers-to-be, she made an appointment with her obstetrician-gynecologist. But unlike many pregnant women, she also contacted a nurse-midwife. "I was getting into natural health and living a natural lifestyle," Kwasa, now 29, explains. "My son's dad, Adé, and I decided we didn't want to have our child in the hospital. I wanted it to be a home experience." Though the first meeting resembled a visit with an ob-gyn when nurse-midwife Nonkululeko Tyehimba, RN, of Harlem took Kwasa's blood pressure, measured her stomach, and used an ultrasound to listen to the baby's heartbeat, the visit differed in significant ways. They talked about Kwasa's diet, herbs she could take like red raspberry, books and videos for her to review, as well as her happiness. "She used to tell me to take walks, have folks cook for me, get lots of pampering," Kwasa recalls. "She was like my mother."

Throughout her pregnancy, Kwasa continued to see Nonkululeko every month in addition to seeing her ob-gyn as a backup.

163

She read books like What to Expect When You're Expecting, *and watched videos depicting women around the world giving birth, which helped her dispel her fears about what was happening to her body. Upon the midwife's suggestion, she oiled her perineum—the area between her vagina and rectum prone to tearing during delivery—with either almond oil, olive oil, or shea butter every day in order to soften and stretch it before delivery. In preparation for the big day, she purchased a variety of supplies (shower curtain, sheets, gauze, etc.) to lie out on her living room floor—the delivery room. When Kwasa's water broke, she called Nonkululeko, who advised her to just sit down and drink some tea. Later, with the father and the midwife present, Kwasa jogged around the apartment to "help bring the baby down." When the pain increased, she simply rocked on the floor while Adé rubbed her back.*

Finally, Kwasa got in her preferred position for delivery—on all fours. "Nonkululeko used to say that [being on] your back is convenient for the doctors but it's not necessarily convenient or comfortable for you, or the easiest way to get the child out of you," Kwasa says. To ease the excruciating pain, she wrapped her arms around her midwife and held for dear life. "I remember that I was just hugging her so hard," she notes. "I was just wailing." When the baby arrived, Adé caught him and handed him to Nonkululeko, who blessed him with an ankh, the Khemetic (Eyptian) symbol for life. Then, the little boy went straight to Kwasa's breast and Adé cut the cord.

Kwasa has no regrets about the way she had her son and would do it again. She feels that an at-home birth with a midwife restores the choices and rights of parents that have been stripped away by the medical establishment's typical way of handling childbirth. "Pregnancy is not a sickness and I feel that's how a lot of folks treat it," she adds. "You're not ill; you're just pregnant." These days she enjoys reading passages from journals she kept during the pregnancy to her now seven-year-old son, Khepera. "He loves it. It's like a fairy tale to him."

The ability to make babies is a wonderful part of our womanhood. It is supposed to be among the most natural events in our lives. But for many of the same reasons black women as a group are at risk for major health problems—poverty, poor access to health care, stressful lifestyles—the road from conception to delivery may be fraught with unanticipated difficulties and challenges. Contrary to stereotypical belief, black women are not fertile Myrtles: One in ten of us will struggle with infertility or the inability to conceive during our childbearing years. While the percentage of black mothers-to-be receiving prenatal care beginning in the first trimester has increased from 60 percent in 1989 to 73 percent in 1998, according to the National Center for Health Statistics, we still lag far behind other groups who receive more timely care. Of all American women, black women have the highest rates of low-birthweight babies (less than 2,500 grams or five and a half pounds), very low-birthweight babies (less than 1,500 grams or two and three-quarter pounds) and infant mortality, or death of a child under one year of age.

Not only are our babies at risk, but we are as well: Black women are four times as likely to die during delivery or after than white women, according to a recent report by the Centers for Disease Control and Prevention. This off-the-charts mortality rate, which usually occurs when pregnancy complications escalate into deaths, affects black women from all socioeconomic groups. It may be due at least in part to the fact that sisters are not in the best health when we get pregnant and tend to receive too little prenatal care and too late.

For these reasons, though pregnancy and childbirth are natural events, we have even more reason than most women to take childbearing very seriously, from the moment we conceive of our offspring in our minds to the moment we hold our cherished one in our arms. To ensure the health of our present and future babies, we must take the very best care of our minds, bodies, and spirits; learn about the process of pregnancy and birth; and explore all of the options before us as mothers-in-the-making.

Making Babies

Planning for a healthy baby starts long before the moment of conception. Some folks give more time and thought to planning a wedding than to bearing a child! We must be sure our minds, bodies, and spirits are prepared to receive this precious gift of life. Following is a checklist of questions to consider.

Six Months to a Year before You Get Pregnant . . .

Prepregnancy checklist

_ Are you in good physical health?

_ Are you in good emotional and spiritual health?

_ If you have high blood pressure or diabetes, is it under control?

_ Are you menstruating regularly?

_ Do you eat a balanced diet of natural foods on most days, and take supplements?

_ Do you exercise most days of the week?

_ Are you at a healthy weight?

_ Are you under any undue stress from a recent life change (loss of a loved one, loss of a job, marriage, a move) or an ongoing life challenge (marital conflict, work difficulty, financial strain)?

_ Are you taking any medications that might interfere with your ability to conceive?

_ Do you work or live in environments that expose you to pollutants or chemicals?

_ Are you prepared financially to get good prenatal care and to raise a child?

_ Is your *partner* healthy physically, emotionally, and spiritually?

If *any* of these questions give you pause, you should take the time to reassess your reasons for wanting a child and the timing. Take steps now to improve your health (Chapters 1 and 2), minimize stress, and get your life in line with your desire to be a mother. Keep reviewing the list of questions until you feel comfortable with your internal responses. Being prepared is one of the greatest gifts you can give to your future baby.

Conscious Conception

At least half of all pregnancies in the United States are unintended or unplanned. Though learning you are pregnant may be a great cause for celebration, for far too many women the news comes as a surprise. The danger in this is that an unprepared mother may put herself and her baby in jeopardy. "When a woman gets pregnant, a lot of the time she doesn't know until the first cycle is missed," says Dr. Thomas "Ken" Taylor, founder of Northwest Women's Care in Roswell, Georgia. "But the first two to eight weeks of pregnancy are the most important. It's when the baby is developing. It's when you can affect the heart muscle, the brain—everything." That is why the experts suggest women who want to get pregnant take folic acid supplements *before* conception in order to prevent potential birth defects that could occur in the early stages of pregnancy.

In other words, having a healthy pregnancy and child is not a given. It requires that we make conscious choices to minimize complications like C-sections and less-than-ideal birth outcomes like prematurity and low birthweight. To women who say, "I didn't plan on getting pregnant," Dr. Taylor responds, "You didn't plan on *not* getting pregnant." In any case, women of childbearing age must be prepared:

Be Physically Active. "A person who is in good shape can go through pregnancy a lot better than one who is not," Dr. Taylor says.

Supplement a Good Diet. With a prenatal multivitamin-mineral pill, get the nutrients you need for a healthy pregnancy, including iron, calcium, and folic acid. Talk to an ob-gyn and/or a nurse-midwife about what you might need.

Reduce Alcohol Intake. Drinking alcohol can inhibit fertility and potentially harm a developing fetus.

Get Regular Checkups. Visit a general provider and an ob-gyn in order to catch any undetected medical problems, including STIs and uncontrolled diabetes or hypertension.

Manage Your Weight. This is not about vanity but health. Obesity has been linked to increased risk of birth defects, pregnancy-induced hypertension, gestational diabetes, Cesarean section, and induced labor, among other poor health outcomes.

Three Months to Six Months *before* You Get Pregnant . . .

Natural Family Planning

Though folks usually think of natural family planning (NFP) as a means of contraception, you can use it as a strategy to boost your chance of conceiving as well. Also referred to as fertility awareness, this process of predicting ovulation also teaches us how to become more aware of and familiar with our bodies, our natural cycles, and the changes that accompany them. In addition to helping us get pregnant, a more intimate relationship with our bodies benefits us in ways that an over-the-counter ovulation predictor kit never can. It also puts us in control of a process that has traditionally been left up to chance or in the hands of doctors.

Natural family planning is not the rhythm method, a less reliable form of contraception that is based on the charting of previous menstrual cycles. To practice natural family planning correctly and effectively, you should first consult an ob-gyn or nurse-midwife for guidance. You'll need to routinely test three factors related to ovulation: (1) the consistency of cervical fluid or discharge, (2) your resting or basal body temperature, and (3) the feel and position of your cervix.

Cervical Fluid. The most reliable sign of ovulation are changes in cervical fluid. We're all familiar with the mucus we see on our panties or wipe away on toilet paper during each month. However, we are probably not as aware of the way this fluid changes in consistency in order to help or hinder sperm transport. Right after our periods end and during the time before and after ovulation, the cervical fluid quality ranges from dry to wet and runny to thick and sticky. It is when the mucus is wet—resembling raw egg whites—that sperm can most easily survive and make their way into the uterus. Each day for two or three months you should take note of the feel of the cervical fluid on your vaginal lips and panties. Record these changes on a calendar or day planner.

Temperature. Though our temperatures usually stay steady at 98.6 degrees Fahrenheit during the day, our temperature upon waking varies during the month in response to a pregnancy-related hormone, progesterone. Before ovulation, waking temperature is about 97 degrees. Upon ovulation, temperature dips slightly, then rises to between 97.6 and 98.6 a day or so later. To get pregnant, you would need to have sexual intercourse on the day your waking temperature drops or before it rises again.

To get an accurate reading, use a basal body thermometer to take your temperature first thing in the morning before you get out of bed, drink, or eat. Record the numbers on a calendar or in your date book for three months before trying to get pregnant in order to get practice and become familiar with your own individual temperature variations. Understand that temperature may also be affected by illness and other factors, so combine this indicator with your testing of cervical fluid.

Other Cervical Changes. Before ovulation, your cervix—a round structure located at the top of your vagina—is typically firm and its opening, or os, is closed. During egg release and after, the cervix rises slightly and softens. The os opens up to allow sperm to enter the uterus freely. To feel your cervix, squat down and stick a finger in your vagina as far as you can reach. Do this before and after ovulation (two weeks after your period begins) for a couple of months until these cervical changes are familiar to you. Record these changes along with your cervical changes and temperature.

To ensure an accurate prediction of ovulation and conception, practice measuring your temperature and cervical changes as long as you need to feel confident. You may also want to combine these methods with the older rhythm method, which predicts ovulation based on previous cycle patterns. Record your cycle length for each of six months: Most women's cycles range from 20 to 35 days. Take the shortest cycle length and subtract 14 days (or the length of the postovulatory phase of your cycle). This number should tell you on what day of your cycle you are likely to ovulate. For further guidance on natural family planning, talk to a gyn or nurse-midwife. Also consult books in Resources.

Pregnancy Barriers

Infertility

After a couple of months of trying, most young, healthy couples expect that they'll be able to conceive a child. But for many—one in ten black women of childbearing age—this quite normal expectation will be met with disappointment, again and again. Infertility is a common problem with many possible causes. A couple is considered infertile after a year of trying with no results. Experts estimate that in 40 percent of cases, the cause of infertility lies with the woman; another 40 percent lies with the man; and 20 percent is unexplained. Common causes include:

Age. After age 35, a woman's production of eggs naturally declines, making it more difficult to conceive. Though most women enter menopause—the stage at which menstruation ceases (see Chapter 10) around age 50—many begin to shift into this stage years earlier, reducing the risk of fertility further still.

Irregular Periods. For a number of reasons including hormonal imbalances, cessation of birth control pills, and stress, some women do not ovulate regularly, which hampers their ability to conceive.

Sexually Transmitted Illnesses (STIs). Common STIs such as chlamydia and gonorrhea can cause scarring of sexual organs in both women and men if they are undetected and left untreated. Such scarring can interfere with the normal process of fertilization. Because these infections may not cause symptoms right away—and because African-Americans tend to have higher rates of STIs—we must have regular gynecological checkups, see our providers if we notice any unusual sores, discharge, or other symptoms, and protect our bodies with condoms. If you suspect you have an STI, see your provider immediately—and tell your partner to do the same.

Pelvic Inflammatory Disease. A result of untreated STIs, pelvic inflammatory disease (PID) can cause serious damage to reproductive organs including the ovaries, the fallopian tubes, and the womb itself. Untreated PID may result in the scarring and twisting of fallopian tubes, hindering ovulation and fertilization. Symptoms of PID include pelvic pain, abnormal bleeding, unusual discharge, and fever. This severe infection must be treated right away.

Other Pelvic Illness. Endometriosis, fibroids, and ovarian cysts may also interfere with conception and implantation of an embryo in your womb. See your doctor annually to detect these problems early. Examine your diet and lifestyle (see Chapters 1, 2, and 7) and make necessary changes in order to heal or at least manage the problems and limit their impact on your fertility.

Sperm Problems. Low sperm counts or sluggish sperm can prevent fertility. Men who are trying to conceive should avoid excessive heat to the genital area caused by wearing tight clothing during intense workouts, and the use of saunas, steam baths, or whirlpools.

Immune System Problems. A woman's cervical fluid must be receptive to sperm in order for them to make a successful trip up the uterus and fallopian tubes. In some cases, the fluid is not of a consistency that will hold sperm; in others, women actually develop antibodies that kill the sperm.

Medical Problems. Certain conditions may hinder fertility. For example, untreated diabetes may affect a woman's cervical fluid, which helps sperm enter the uterus.

Alcohol and Drugs. Drinking alcohol frequently triggers hormonal changes that make it difficult for both women and men to conceive, and may cause sexual dysfunction.

Stress. The catch-all cause of many health challenges, chronic or excessive stress may inhibit the sexual function and normal reproductive processes of either sex. The inability to conceive itself can cause great anxiety. Women participating in a mind-body infertility program at Harvard Medical School's Division of Behavioral Medicine that emphasizes stress-reducing mind-body activities (meditation, yoga, social support) significantly increased their rate of conception, indicating that the impact of stress on fertility is real.

To Naturally Improve Your Chances of Conceiving a Healthy Child

Lifestyle. Get a physical with a fertility expert to rule out any medical problems. Practice fertility awareness with the help of a family planning counselor or your ob-gyn to increase your chance of conception. Aim to have sex the day of ovulation (approximately two weeks after the first day of your period) and a couple days after. Use these opportunities to really enhance lovemaking and orgasm—the contractions help facilitate conception.

Nutrition. Avoid processed foods which may affect your hormones and overall health. Replace them with a variety of fresh produce, whole grains, and plant proteins.

Supplements/Herbs. You should already be taking prenatal vitamins with folic acid. Extra vitamin C and zinc may help.

Mind-body Methods. Express and examine your feelings about your difficulty conceiving through journaling, joining a support group, or talking to a mental health professional trained in helping individuals cope with infertility. Regularly practice your relaxation technique of choice (meditation, deep breathing, visualization) to ease stress.

Hands-On Healing. In some cases, chiropractic care can correct misalignments in the pelvis that hamper fertility.

Miscarriage

For many women the joy of getting pregnant is dashed by the heartbreak of miscarriage, which occurs most often during the first three months of pregnancy. The possible reasons for miscarriage are multiple, including the age of the mother, hormonal imbalance, STIs, pelvic illness, and immune system problems as described above. Emotional problems and conflicts about motherhood may also contribute to miscarriages. In this case, you will need to work closely with your ob-gyn, certified nurse-midwife, or a fertility specialist to identify the problem and improve your chances of bringing a child to term.

Self-Awareness Tool

Great Expectations

Being pregnant and becoming a mother are supposed to be among of the greatest joys of being a woman. But in reality, along with our hopes come some fears about what will happen to our bodies, how we will get through labor, and how our lives will change once a child has arrived. Your state of mind before, during, and after pregnancy is key to your own well-being and that of your child. Don't bury fears or ambivalence; get information and support instead. Begin by writing responses to these questions.

What do I fear most about being pregnant/becoming a mother?

_____

_____

_____

_____

_____

What excites me most about being pregnant/becoming a mother?

_____

_____

_____

_____

_____

The Adoption Option

There are many reasons to consider adopting a child—infertility, advanced age, the desire to help a disadvantaged child, or perhaps you're single and you'd like to be a mother. More than half of the children in America waiting to be adopted are African-American, and the waiting period for adopting black and mixed-race children is typically half that for white children. Learn more by contacting an attorney specializing in adoption or call your local department of social services. The following organizations can also provide facts: the National Adoption Center (800-TO-ADOPT); the Black Adoption Consortium (800-552-0222); and the Black Adoption Placement and Research Center (510-839-3678).

Being Pregnant

Morning sickness, rounded bellies, swollen ankles, kicking babies—all signs of the joys and pains of pregnancy. We may look upon this time in our lives with a mixture of pleasure, fear, and amazement, knowing full well that something quite powerful and miraculous is occurring within us as we create life. It is an awesome time during which we must treat our bodies and our responsibility as mothers reverently and respectfully.

Despite what the medical establishment might have us believe, our bodies in their healthiest state are equipped to bring a healthy baby to term naturally. But given that black women are more likely than others to have problems—from gestational diabetes to pre-eclampsia (hypertension during pregnancy), we must take extra special care of ourselves and our babies throughout gestation.

One of the most important steps is establishing a relationship with an obstetrician-gynecologist and/or a certified nurse-midwife that you feel comfortable with and who supports your desire to lead a natural lifestyle and have a natural pregnancy. The next is to see the caregiver regularly—even when you are feeling good. An ob-gyn or midwife can detect any problems that might crop up, such as excessive weight gain or a rise in blood pressure, and help you manage them before they affect your pregnancy. Your provider can also help you minimize any complications that might result from preexisting diabetes or hypertension. (If you do not know of any midwives in your community, check with your ob-gyn or local hospital. See also the Resources.)

Trimester by Trimester

0 to 3 months

Lifestyle. Continue to get physical activity in regularly through low-impact activities such as walking or swimming. Give yourself more time to rest and sleep.

Nutrition. Make sure you are eating a balanced diet of natural foods including fresh vegetables, fruit, grains, and plant proteins. Eat as you normally would—no more food and no less. If you have morning sickness during this period, eat smaller, more frequent meals and drink plenty of water. Eliminate all alcohol and caffeine.

Supplements/Herbs. Talk to your ob-gyn and/or nurse-midwife about which supplements you may need. Iron and calcium are typically recommended. High doses of vitamins A, C, and D may be toxic to your baby. Certain herbs like ginger or red raspberry for morning sickness may be safe to take during pregnancy but do not take any herbs without consulting your ob-gyn or certified nurse-midwife.

Mind-body Methods. To cope with mood swings which are common at this time, try writing in a journal or indulging in a relaxing hobby once a day. Talk to other expectant mothers or current mothers to get support and advice. If you need, let yourself have a good cry.

4 to 6 Months

Lifestyle. Continue moderate exercise to stay strong and prevent excessive weight gain.

Nutrition. Continue eating a balanced diet with an emphasis on fiber-rich foods to relieve constipation.

Supplements/Herbs. If you have not already, talk to your ob-gyn and/or nurse-midwife about which supplements you may need such as iron and calcium.

Mind-Body Methods. Yoga is a gentle way to stay limber and ease pain while pregnant.

Hands-On Healing. Massage may help if you experience back pain, leg swelling, or varicose veins.

7 to 9 Months

Lifestyle. Getting sufficient rest may be a challenge now with the back pain and the urgency to go to the bathroom that often occurs during this time. So slow down and take it easy.

Nutrition. Fill up on fruit and vegetable juices if you suffer heartburn or constipation.

Supplements/Herbs. If you have not already, talk to your ob-gyn and/or nurse-midwife about which supplements you may need such as iron and calcium.

Mind-Body Methods. Try deep breathing to relieve headaches and for relaxation.

During the first four months, you should see your ob-gyn or nurse-midwife once a month, and more frequently after that, if your pregnancy is normal. If your pregnancy is considered high risk, your provider will tell you how often to come in for checkups. To be safe, keep all of your prenatal appointments, follow your provider's advice, and call if you notice any changes in your health.

Giving Birth

When we think of childbirth, we can all probably bring to mind images of a woman lying in a hospital bed writhing in pain as a male doctor cajoles her to "push!" This familiar image has inspired fear in the hearts of many women, who dread the pain and the unpredictability of childbirth. But the medical version of this natural experience is not the only one. These days, mothers have a number of choices in terms of where and how to have their babies. If you have an uncomplicated or low-risk pregnancy, here are just a few options:

Natural Birth Environments

At-Home Birth. With the help of a certified nurse-midwife, having your baby at home can be preferable for many reasons. You are in an environment familiar to you, you can have as many family members and friends around as you want, and you—and your little one—can recover at home as well. A nurse-midwife can counsel you in how to prepare your home environment, supplies you need, and what to do in case of an emergency. See the Resources for where to get information on home births.

Birthing Rooms and Centers. Whether in a hospital or separate facility, birthing rooms are an increasingly popular option among mothers. Like your own home, birthing rooms offer a comfortable environment in which you can bring personal items, and a number of family members and friends. A nurse-midwife assists in your natural birth process—minus medical equipment and drugs. But you have the advantage of having medical equipment nearby if needed. During recovery, your new baby may share the room with you as opposed to sleeping in a separate nursery.

Underwater Births. In utero, babies live in water, receiving oxygen from their mothers. Underwater births allow them to leave this protective cocoon and enter a similar environment before emerging into the world to take their first breath. Certain hospitals offer it as an option, though it is not usually covered by insurance.

Natural Helpers

Midwives. Once as likely to deliver babies as doctors, midwives have long been serving the black community. Midwives don't only offer experience with bringing babies into the world and training; they also often provide more time, attention, and support than ob-gyns. They also base their practice on the belief that pregnancy and childbirth are natural events. There are generally two types: *certified nurse-midwives* (CNMs), who are trained in nursing and midwifery; and *lay midwives,* who typically have more experience than formal training.

CNMs may be preferable because of their training and because they are often affiliated with an ob-gyn or a group of doctors. But as with any health provider, your comfort with the provider and her methods is key. Once you've contacted a midwife, be sure to ask questions about her years of experience and training, the number of healthy babies she's delivered, procedures in case of emergencies, and fees.

Doulas. Another practice that dates back centuries is labor support. Doulas, also called birth assistants, are women who offer care and support during labor and delivery. Like midwives, doulas provide more than advice; they respond to a laboring woman's needs and "mother" her throughout the process of birth. The presence of a doula may decrease the need for pain medication, shorten labor, and lower the risk of a C-section. Doulas can work well with midwives or doctors. To find one, ask your midwife or doctor for referrals or see the Resources.

Natural Childbirth

A number of natural childbirth methods allows women to reduce the pain and discomfort of pregnancy while also avoiding pain relief medications that may affect the baby. The Lamaze method is most well known, but there are a few others that all educate women about the process of labor and delivery while also providing them with relaxation techniques to minimize the pain of childbirth. To learn these methods, you and your mate can attend childbirth education classes around the seventh month of pregnancy. In class you'll learn about what happens to your body during labor, and how to use breathing and other techniques to cope with labor pains. Your mate learns how to support and assist you through the process. To find a class, ask your midwife or doctor for referrals.

Breastfeeding: Nature's Formula

The myths and wives' tales about breastfeeding are many—it ruins your figure and causes breasts to sag, it makes your baby become too attached to you, and you must drink milk to produce it. These beliefs are false, and the benefits of breastfeeding outweight any mild discomfort and inconvenience a nursing mother may experience. Experts have long known that breastmilk ensures an infant's proper development and even wards off infection. In recent years, studies have indicated that breast-fed babies developed a higher IQ and might be less likely to die from sudden infant death syndrome, or SIDS, than bottle-fed babies. Unfortunately, only 27 percent of African-American mothers breastfeed, even though our children are often born premature with low birthweight, and succumb disproportionately to SIDS (see below). To learn more about breastfeeding, contact La Leche League (800-638-6607).

SIDS: Our Babies Are More Prone

Once known as crib death, sudden infant death syndrome (SIDS) is a medical disorder whose cause is unknown. It occurs during sleep without warning to seemingly healthy infants, and claims about 3,000 one-week to twelve-month-old babies each year in the United States. SIDS is the leading cause of death for that age group. African-American babies are more than twice as likely to succumb to SIDS than white babies. To prevent it, don't smoke during or after pregnancy, have your baby nap and sleep on her back, and use a firm mattress in a safety approved crib. For more facts on SIDS, contact the Sudden Infant Death Syndrome Alliance (800-221-7437) and the National Center for the Prevention of SIDS (800-638-7437).

Resources

American College of Nurse-Midwives, 818 Connecticut Avenue, NW, Suite 900, Washington, DC 20006.

American Society for Reproductive Medicine, 1209 Montgomery Highway, Birmingham, AL 35216-2809.

Association for Childbirth at Home International, PO Box 430, Glendale, CA 91209.

Doulas of America, 13513 North Grove Drive, Alpine, UT 84004.

March of Dimes, 1275 Mamaroneck Avenue, White Plains, NY 10605.

National Family Planning and Reproductive Health Association, 122 C Street, NW, Suite 380, Washington, DC 20001.

Planned Parenthood Federation of America, 810 Seventh Avenue, New York, NY 10019; www.plannedparenthood.org.

Pregnancy and Infant Loss Center, 1421 East Wayzata Boulevard, Wayzata, MN 55391.

The Traditional Childbearing Group, PO Box 638, Boston, MA 02118.

Having Your Baby: A Guide for African-American Women, by Hilda Hutcherson MD (Ballantine).

Healing Mind, Healthy Woman: Using the Mind-Body Connection to Manage Stress and Take Control of Your Life, by Alice Domar (Delta).

Planning for Pregnancy, Birth and Beyond, by the American College of Obstetricians and Gynecologists (ACOG).

Pregnancy Nutrition: Good Health for You and Your Baby, by Elizabeth M. Ward (Wiley).

What to Expect When You're Experiencing Infertility: How to Cope with the Emotional Crisis and Survive, by Debby Peoples and Harriette Rovner Ferguson, CSW (Norton & Co.).

Chapter 10

~

Time for the Change: Menopause

NATURAL WOMAN: DR. YVONNE LEWIS, ND

While in her late thirties, Dr. Yvonne Lewis, a lifestyle consultant residing in Arlington, Texas, started to experience mild bouts of depression and forgetfulness. At first, she figured it was all due to stress. But after talking to girlfriends who were complaining about skipped periods and feeling "hot," Yvonne thought that her symptoms and those of her friends were probably due to menopause. She did some reading on the subject and realized she had in fact entered the "change of life."

Having been raised a health-conscious Seventh-Day Adventist, Yvonne never considered anything but natural solutions to her symptoms. She eats a vegetarian diet and takes supplements containing fiber, vitamins, minerals, and other nutrients. She swears by her daily cups of garden sage tea as a remedy for night sweats. To keep from forgetting important details such as people's names, for example, Yvonne has learned to associate each person's name with a physical characteristic. And to keep the rest of life's details in focus, "you make lists," she advises. "You leave yourself notes and you have checklists of things to do."

In her effort to stay challenged mentally, Yvonne also went back to school to get a degree in naturopathy, a health care practice that emphasizes natural remedies. "You should never just throw up your hands and say, 'Well, I can't do this because I'm too old,'" she adds. "You just keep working at whatever you do and becoming the best at whatever you do." Now the author of a self-published book on menopause called Where's the Toast?, *Yvonne makes an effort to focus on the positive aspects of midlife. In addition to saying good-bye forever to periods and pads, Yvonne says: "I think that there is a wisdom that accompanies this time of life and a self-knowledge that is really unparalleled. We are much more aware of who we are and where we're going. It's a really good time for knowing yourself, for mentoring, for really finding out, really knowing who you are. I also think that it's a good time for doing a lot for others. You have some free time to be of greater service to community, your church." Yvonne's relationship with her Lord is also a fundamental source of her optimism and strength.*

Meaning pause of menses or menstruation, menopause is not an event but a transitional period in a woman's life triggered by natural hormonal changes. Known commonly as "the change of life," menopause typically includes three phases: perimenopause, menopause, and postmenopause. These medical terms describe a process that begins with skipped periods and is defined by your very last period. Also known as the climacteric, this process usually starts in the mid- to late forties, lasting from five to ten years or longer.

But menopause is not just a physical happening; it is a spiritual and emotional one, too. More "change" may be going on than a few hot flashes. Some sisters find themselves in the throws of mood swings and insecurities they have not encountered since adolescence. Some sisters look back on their lives and their youth with a sense of loss and regret. Yet others say good-bye to their childbearing years gleefully while looking forward to living the future on their own terms.

Wherever menopause finds you, know that you are undergoing a remarkable metamorphosis, that is, a "change in physical form . . . or substance," according to one dictionary. Just like any other stage in life, this one may require some reassessment, shedding of the old, and embracing the new. Instead of despairing as Western culture expects women to do, consider taking a more purposeful and powerful stance: *Menopause is here. What will you do with it?*

Natural Healing Is Our History

Clearly women of all cultures go through menopause, but not all women experience it in the same way. The traditional culture of our West African foremothers and contemporaries offers a perspective that can help us enter menopause joyfully and gracefully. In indigenous African cultures, elders are well respected for their knowledge and life experiences. According to Malidoma Patrice Somé, because age connotes maturity and wisdom among traditional Africans such as the Dagara people of Burkina Faso, people actually look forward to getting older. Age also brings traditional people closer to the place where their ancestors reside and to the spirit world. To be "old" is to be almost sacred. To be old is to be powerful. This is also true of the !Kung women in southern Africa, who don't have a word for "hot flash" in their language.

This positive attitude toward aging has largely survived in our community. Who doesn't have a grandma or an aunt whom we rely on for guidance and support? If not a relative, we look to an older neighbor or church or mosque member. Our elder women are powerful women—not simply frail or crazy. We look upon their usually wrinkle-free faces (Black don't crack!) and see the wisdom and strength of generations in their eyes. We listen to their stories and marvel at what they have survived. Who would not want to be filled with their grace, their fortitude, their authority?

As you rethink your ideas about getting older and prepare for the pause, it might help to engage in another Africanism: seeking advice and counsel from elder women. Find out what menopause was like

185

for your mother, aunt, grandmother. Benefit from the fact that menopause is no longer a taboo topic and ask plenty of questions. Then share your knowledge and wisdom with others. As you become more aware of physical changes that accompany the change and learn more about your body, trade tales with other women your age and younger women, too. Support and celebrate each other in your transition.

Very little research exists on African-American women and menopause, but a few small studies have shown that, as compared to white women of the same age, sisters going through the change are more likely to perceive it as a natural event—not a calamity. Black women also prefer to use natural remedies, including herbs and vitamin supplements, to alleviate symptoms rather than the standard medical therapy, hormone replacement. Perhaps this is due as much to our heritage and more positive attitude toward aging as it is to our distrust of pills and the medical establishment.

Top Ten Benefits of Midlife Changes

Youth isn't everything. Here's what you have to be thankful for:

- No more pregnancy worries or need for contraception
- No more periods or PMS
- Lower risk of fibroids; existing fibroids may shrink
- Greater wisdom
- More time with your partner
- Stronger sense of self and independence
- More time for friendships
- Freedom to explore hobbies and travel
- Opportunity to focus on career
- More financial security

What's Going On? Understanding the Change

The phenomenon we call menopause is a slow process that takes several years to unfold. It is marked by a number of signs and symptoms that experts have categorized into specific phases.

Perimenopause (Approximately Ages 35 to 45)

In our mid-forties and sometimes earlier, women begin to have irregular menstrual cycles or skipped periods. This is due to the fact that our ovaries are beginning to produce less estrogen and other hormones including progesterone. No one knows why this occurs but perimenopause marks the gradual shift from our childbearing years to menopause. During this period, women may experience related physical and psychological changes, including hot flashes, memory loss, anxiety and mood swings, among others. If you have had PMS, you are more likely to experience symptoms during perimenopause. Other women sail through this transition with nothing more than bleeding irregularities. A fundamental change is underway.

Menopause (Approximately Ages 45 to 55)

In our early fifties, women's periods cease altogether. You may reach menopause around the same time your mother did. We know we have completed menopause when we've had no period for an entire year. At this point, pregnancy is no longer possible (without medical intervention). The amounts of estrogen and other hormones being produced by the ovaries have dropped off sharply though not completely. In fact, estrogen and other key hormones—progesterone, testosterone, and DHEA—continue to flow from other sources such as the adrenal glands (above the kidneys), pineal gland in the brain, and body fat. The balance of these shifting hormones—and the effects on quality of life and health—varies from woman to woman.

Many natural healers suspect that while menopause is natural, menopausal symptoms are not. Acupuncturist and herbalist Beverly Coleman, who resides in Sedona, Arizona, believes that at least some of the problems women face stem from poor function of the kidney meridian or energy system (see Chapter six). "In other cultures, it's the kidney that is the captain of hormonal activity and of the body's 'fire,' " she explains. "When the kidneys become deficient, the body waters don't function well and the person overheats." The kidneys can age prematurely, she says, because of stress and poor diet—too much salt and acid-forming foods like sugar. She also suggests that because the feminine identity of "post-slave" women has been so violated, we have greater difficulty with "female" problems. "We're culturally violated in that our concepts of beauty, of what it is to be a woman, are perverted in slave culture," she explains. The answer is acceptance. "When you find women who just love themselves, love being women, love their position with men, these women really have much less trouble [with menopause]," she notes.

Whatever the cause or causes, menopausal symptoms are quite real. The decrease in hormones may trigger a variety of changes, including skin temperature fluctuations or hot flashes, the thinning of vaginal walls and drying of vaginal fluids, and cognitive impairments including short-term memory lags and concentration difficulties. Bone mass typically decreases rapidly at this time—though most black women start off with greater bone density than white or Asian women. A woman's risk of developing heart disease begins to rival that of a man. Hot flashes are the most common complaint of menopausal women who have symptoms.

Postmenopause (Approximately Age 55 and beyond)

At this point, the body still produces hormones but at much lower levels. While the risk of getting pregnant and the need for birth control are behind us, other health issues may emerge. Fractures of the hip, wrist, and spine—the consequence of bone loss and other factors—are more common during postmenopause. The risk of developing heart disease rises for women, particularly those with risk factors such as obesity, poor nutrition, physical inactivity, hypertension, diabetes, or a family history of heart disease. Because of these factors, and poor access to good health care, black women ages 35 to 74 have a 72 percent higher death rate from heart disease than white women.

Early Menopause

A woman may enter menopause earlier than expected for a number of reasons:

Surgery. Hysterectomy, or removal of the uterus and often the ovaries (known as oophorectomy) to treat reproductive disorders such as fibroids or endometriosis, will result in an artificial menopause. In this case, hormone levels drop abruptly, possibly making symptoms worse than they would be otherwise. Removing the uterus alone will cause a less dramatic and temporary decline in reproductive hormones.

Cancer Treatment. Chemotherapy for cancer may also cause a woman to enter menopause before her time. This permanent side effect is more likely to occur the older a woman is when she received chemotherapy.

Immune System Problems. For unknown reasons, some women develop a condition in which their body makes antibodies that attack the ovaries, causing them to function improperly and produce fewer hormones.

Self-Awareness Tool

Take a Pause

Health problems in midlife are not inevitable. Whatever stage you are in—perimenopause, menopause, or postmenopause—take the opportunity to examine your lifestyle and state of mind-body-spirit health, and make any necessary changes.

- How often do you exercise? Does your routine include strength or resistance training to increase bone health?
- Is your diet based mainly on fresh, natural foods such as vegetables, fruits, and whole grains? Do you often eat more or less than you need to feel satisfied?
- Do you take nutritional supplements?
- Do you often feel "stressed out"? What do you do to relax?
- What efforts do you make to grow mentally/intellectually? Have you learned anything new lately?
- Whom do you rely on for support and companionship? Do you feel loved—or lonely?
- Are you happy? Do you have any deferred dreams yet to fulfill?
- Do you have spiritual or moral beliefs that reassure you and guide your life?

NATURAL WOMAN: MONICA KAUFMAN

Monica Kaufman, a television news anchor based in Atlanta, was already perimenopausal when she had her uterus and ovaries removed to treat a case of endometriosis. The hot flashes were more than the 45-year-old could take, so she went to her doctor, who raised a concern about heart disease and osteoporosis—two conditions that affect women more commonly after menopause. Monica, who was reluctant to take any medicine, tried hormone replacement therapy (HRT) for about three months. She started to gain weight in spite of her three-day-a-week exercise program. So she stopped taking the HRT and decided instead to do some research at the library, in bookstores and in health food stores. This led her to create a special news program on the topic, called "Hot Flash: The Truth About Menopause." It was one of the highest-rated shows in her station's history.

To treat her symptoms, which also included mood swings and vaginal dryness, Monica experimented with several natural remedies including vitamin E, herbal teas, and soy supplements. She increased the amount of soy foods in her diet, including soy milk and even soy ice cream! Today, she is glad she ceased the hormonal ther-

apy. In October 1998, Monica was diagnosed with early-stage breast cancer. Her physician removed the cancerous cells, which were the type that feed on estrogen. Though she is not yet considered cancer free, in terms of her decision to stop taking estrogen replacement therapy, Monica says, "I'm glad I listened to my senses."

These days she continues to exercise frequently, either with a trainer at the gym or by walking on her own. She recently decided to give up dairy products, which her body can no longer tolerate. Monica also continues to speak out about menopause, whether she is traveling on assignment or talking to friends or new acquaintances. "I believe in girl talk," she notes. "You have to talk to other women about it as well as your physician." To cope with physical symptoms, she stresses diet, supplements, and exercise. To adjust to aging, she advises women to celebrate their maturity. "Some women mourn the loss of fertility, but you've done that," Monica says. "[Menopause] is God's way of saying, 'Well done, girl. Here's your break.'"

Natural Solutions to Ten Common Menopause Signs

Hot Flashes/Night Sweats

These sudden and intense waves of heat that cause women to perspire even in a cool room are triggered by fluctuations in the body's natural cooling system. They typically begin in the chest or neck and travel upward but you may feel them all over. Many women also experience a racing heartbeat, flushed skin, and dizziness for a few minutes. Sometimes referred to as "power surges," hot flashes are unpredictable and may be embarrassing.

Lifestyle. Exercise regularly; dress in layers.

Nutrition. Drink eight or more glasses of water per day. Eating more food containing phytoestrogens (plant estrogens)—soy products (soymilk, tofu, miso, tempeh), yams, nuts—may help offset hormonal imbalance. Be sure to choose sugar-free soymilk, says Coleman. Eliminate all sources of caffeine and avoid alcohol, which may exacerbate flashes. Women who have a taste for hot or spicy foods may have to limit or avoid them.

Supplements/Herbs. For improved kidney function, Coleman recommends herbs such as parsley, juniper berries, and nettles. She suggests visiting the local herb store for formulas designed for women. Natural progesterone supplements or wild yam cream may also help women whose bodies produce too little progesterone. Vitamin E, evening primrose oil, dong quai, ginseng, black cohosh, and homeopathic remedies may also be helpful.

Mind-Body Methods. Make efforts to face and heal negative emotions such as anger and fear. And don't sweat the small stuff. "Anyone will tell you that they'll get more flashes when they're upset," says Coleman. She recommends reading the work of personal growth expert Iyanla Vanzant to find peace.

Hands-On Healing. Acupressure or acupuncture may help.

Insomnia

The inability to fall and stay asleep during this time may be related to hot flashes and other midlife changes.

Lifestyle. Regular exercise can minimize fatigue and deepen sleep.

Nutrition. Avoid eating late at night. Eliminate all sources of caffeine and avoid alcohol.

Supplements/Herbs. Herbs such as valerian (as a tea) and lavendar (in a bath) may help you unwind before sleeping.

Mind-Body Methods. Sometimes we sleep poorly because we take worries to bed with us. Minimize stress through routine meditation or deep breathing.

Vaginal Dryness

The decrease in estrogen causes the vaginal walls to thin and become dryer, often leading to painful intercourse and increased bacterial infections.

Supplements/Herbs. The herb black cohosh may help thicken vaginal walls much like estrogen does; consult a licensed herbalist for recommendations.

Low Libido

Due to either a decline in testosterone, the pain of vaginal dryness, or a lack of energy or sexual interest, many menopausal women's sex lives slow down.

Lifestyle. Regular exercise will increase energy and improve body image for those whose libido problems are related to fatigue, weight gain, or fears of aging. Sometimes having more sex—not less—with the help of lubricants can boost sex drive. Experimentation with the help of educational sex videos may also help.

Supplements/Herbs. The hormone DHEA may boost sex drive in women who are deficient in it. Homeopathy may also help.

Hands-On Healing. Try acupuncture.

Moodiness

Much like PMS, menopausal mood swings may cause women to feel unexplicably sad or more sensitive than usual. These emotional ups and downs may be triggered by hormonal changes or they may be due to the stress of disappointments or unmet needs and expectations that emerge at midlife.

Lifestyle. Routine exercise provides a natural mood boost.

Nutrition. A balanced diet low in processed, unnatural foods will support balanced moods. Eliminate all sources of caffeine and avoid alcohol, which alter mood.

Supplements/Herbs. Herbs such as St. John's wort improve mood swings. Homeopathic remedies may also help.

Mind-Body Methods. Express your emotions and reduce stress through journaling, a menopause support group, or therapy. If mood swings are severe and leave you feeling blue for longer than two weeks, see a therapist for counseling.

Hands-On Healing. Acupuncture may help.

Nervousness

Many menopausal women complain about feeling anxious and worried more than in the past. The cause of this symptom is not clear but it is quite common.

Supplements/Herbs. Anxiety-reducing herbs include St. John's wort and valerian.

Mind-Body Methods. Meditation and yoga help calm the mind and spirit. If anxiety is extreme, you may want to discuss the causes with a therapist.

Hands-On Healing. Massage and reflexology may be especially helpful for deep relaxation.

Fuzzy Thinking/Memory Loss

A common concern of menopausal women, "fuzzy thinking" or an inability to focus and recall information is not necessarily a sign of severe mental decline or dementia as many women fear. These symptoms are most likely due to normal changes that you can offset through natural means.

Lifestyle. Exercise increases blood flow and oxygen to the brain, improving its function.

Nutrition. A balanced, nutrient-filled diet that supports optimum memory.

Supplements/Herbs. Herbs like ginkgo biloba and ginseng may help; consult a licensed practitioner.

Mind-Body Methods. Excessive stress can interfere with normal brain function. Mind-body activities like yoga or meditation can reduce stress and improve your ability to concentrate.

Bone Loss

Our bone density decreases throughout our lives but bone loss accelerates during perimenopause and menopause. Health experts and medical doctors often focus on calcium—particularly from milk and dairy products, which many blacks can't tolerate—but several factors influence bone health. You can protect your bones through a variety of natural means.

Lifestyle. Routine exercise, including weight or resistance training (free weights, weight machines, resistance bands), strengthens not only the bones themselves, but the muscles and joints, decreasing the risk of falls and fractures.

Nutrition. A balanced diet high in fresh produce and other plant foods and low in processed foods. Avoid caffeine and alcohol.

Supplements/Herbs. In addition to a multivitamin-mineral supplement, extra calcium, vitamin D, vitamin C and magnesium will help protect bones.

Hands-On Healing. Chiropractic may help maintain bone health through realignment of the spine.

Depression and Menopause

Menopause does not cause clinical depression, a persistent serious mental illness requiring treatment. Still, many women going through the change of life have bouts of anxiety, irritability, anger, and sadness. Fluctuating hormones, especially declining levels of estrogen, may be a factor, but women in midlife are often dealing with life stressors—including changes in their own health status or body image, the illness or death of parents, the departure of children, loss of a partner, and retirement—that can wreak emotional havoc. If you suspect your mood changes are temporary and related to one of these life circumstances, you can try lifting your spirits by exercising regularly, relaxing through meditation or massage, focusing your attention on a new hobby or project or getting together with friends for support. However, if your blue mood lasts for longer than two weeks, contact a therapist (see Chapter 14).

NATURAL WOMAN: BETTY ROBINSON

Fate brought Betty Robinson to the chiropractor's table in June 1999. Although the 43-year-old college program coordinator had been curious about chiropractic medicine for some time, she was discouraged by the cost. Then at a free screening offered at a local cultural event, Betty found a reason to reconsider. "The X rays revealed that I had a curve in my spinal column," she says. Betty's bones had begun the process of degeneration. If the curve in her spine was left untreated, it could eventually develop into osteoporosis.

Betty began seeing Montclair, New Jersey, chiropractor Alfred Davis, three times a week. Dr. Davis applied pressure to Betty's joints, working to restore proper alignment of her spine. After just a few sessions, Betty saw a definite improvement. "Stress at my job would cause the muscles in my neck and shoulders to tighten," she explains. "I tried self-massage and even went to a masseuse. Nothing seemed to help." Dr. Davis was able to work out the knots and teach Betty proper methods to position herself during daily activities including exercise.

She was surprised by the positive effects that chiropractic care also had on other health problems. "My sessions with Dr. Davis re-

196

lieved my headaches and even helped drain my sinuses," she adds. Along with vitamin and mineral supplements, Betty maintains a diet based on fresh fruits and vegetables. After five months of treatment, she has minimized the threat of osteoporosis naturally.

Where's My Waist? Weight Gain at Midlife

Keeping the pounds at bay doesn't get easier after age 35. The natural aging process gradually reduces muscle—the most efficient calorie-burning tissue—as well as aerobic fitness and metabolism. Many of us become less active. While experts aren't sure what effect menopause has on weight gain, women's tendency to accumulate fat around their waistline by age 50 may be a result of falling estrogen levels. The problem is the weight not only doesn't look cute, but also increases our risk of heart disease and other health challenges.

The best way to reverse the accumulation of pounds is to keep moving. Maximize your metabolism by doing aerobic exercise such as walking, swimming, or dancing three to five days a week for 20 to 60 minutes. Also key is strength-training exercise, using weight or resistance, 2 or 3 times a week to build muscle. And watch what you eat, but avoid dieting. Commit to a natural balanced diet, smaller portions, and less fat and sugar.

Resources

North American Menopause Society, PO Box 94527, Cleveland, OH 44101-4527.

Older Women's League, 666 Eleventh Street, NW, Suite 700, Washington, DC 20001.

ᴜve's Hormone Book: Making Informed Choices About ᴜse, by Susan M. Love, MD, with Karen Lindsey (Random ᴐ).

ood and Our Bones: The Natural Way to Prevent Osteoporosis, by Annemarie Colbin (Plume).

Menopausal Years: The Wise Woman Way: Alternative Approaches for Women 30-90, by Susan S. Weed (Ash Tree).

The Perimenopause Handbook: What Every Woman Needs to Know About the Years Before Menopause, by Carol Turkington and Susan Johnson (Contemporary Books).

What Your Doctor May Not Tell You About Menopause: The Breakthrough Book on Natural Progesterone, by John R. Lee, MD, and Virginia L. Hopkins (Warner Books).

Where's the Toast? A Woman's Guide to Managing Menopause Naturally, by Yvonne Lewis-Booth (Renew Publishing).

Chapter 11

~

Living with Lupus

NATURAL WOMAN: DEBRA M. ROLON

When Debra Rolon first started to feel more fatigued than normal when she was only 20 years old, she chalked it up to the stress of planning her wedding. But over time, the tiredness continued and she also started to develop headaches as well as concentration problems at work. By the following year, 1985, the executive secretary couldn't pull herself out of bed some days. Her arm swelled up and her hair started falling out. "As the symptoms got more bizarre, I decided to consult a doctor," she recalls. Her physician believed she had rheumatoid arthritis. However, when Debra's condition worsened later that year, and she suffered symptoms such as poor appetite and frequent fevers, she went to the ER and learned she had lupus.

"I was bewildered," she says. "I had never heard of lupus." Soon she would know the disease like the back of her hand. "I immediately started doing research on it," she recalls, contacting the Lupus Foundation of America (see the Resources) and getting information from her doctor. She chose to eat a more balanced diet, includ-

*ing fresh fruits, vegetables, calcium-rich foods to counteract the ef-
fect of medication (prednisone and Imuran) on her bones, and
olive oil for joint pain. "One of the things with lupus is that you suffer from extreme fatigue," Debra explains. "Making changes in my
diet helped my energy level. And I don't suffer as many joint pains
as I did previously."*

*Debra's health was sound enough for her to go on and have two
successful pregnancies in spite of the fact that women with lupus
were once advised against having babies. During each pregnancy
she maintained a healthy diet, exercised with tapes, and made sure
to get enough rest. She hasn't suffered a flare-up of symptoms in
nearly a decade. Not letting herself get stressed and staying positive
are the secrets of her success. "In the beginning, I had the old* Why
me? *attitude," Debra says. "I fought against it a lot. But with lupus,
that doesn't work. I had to embrace it. Learn all I could about it.
Accept that it's now part of me. Live with it and work side by side
with it. When I started doing that, things became easier. If I have to
cancel plans, rather than getting upset, I realize it's a process I have
to go through. It's necessary for me to take care of myself."*

It has a strange name and strange symptoms. Meaning "wolf" in
Latin, lupus is a condition in which the body's natural defense mech-
anism—the immune system—turns against the body's own tissues,
causing mild to severe symptoms. It's a disease with a poorly understood cause and unpredictable progression in each individual. The
bad news about lupus is that there is no cure. The good news is that
the disease often goes into remission, periods in which all signs of illness abate, and a woman with lupus can lead an active and full life.

Lupus is a disease with a black female face. It affects women more
often than men and African-Americans more often than whites.
According to some estimates, 1 in every 250 sisters, typically between
the ages of 15 and 44, will get lupus, but the number may be even
higher. (It is also more common in women of Native American,
Asian, and Hispanic descent than among white women.) Again, no
one understands why. One University of Alabama at Birmingham
study comparing African-American, Hispanic, and Caucasian people

with lupus recently found that black and Hispanic lupus patients got the disease at a younger age than white patients and had more "active" disease—more symptoms more often. Blacks with lupus are also more likely to develop kidney disease than nonblacks.

Because of its potential severity and unpredictable nature, lupus can have as a detrimental effect on our emotions and spirits as it can have on our bodies. Those learning to cope with lupus must understand that their mental state, relationships, careers, and financial stability, as well as their health, are all at stake.

Women may not be able to control the onset of lupus, but they can control their experience with it. If you have lupus, you should take steps to prevent the worsening of symptoms, and maintain a positive attitude. In talking about chronic conditions like lupus, people often use words like "fighting," "battle," and "killer." It may be more helpful to think in terms of *living with* the disease day to day. Instead of a battle that you could win or lose, think of your life with lupus as an onward march.

Lupus Lowdown

Misconceptions about lupus contribute to unnecessary fears. What you should know:

Myth: Lupus is a death sentence.
Fact: No longer. With proper care, most people with lupus can live as long as those without it.

Myth: Lupus is AIDS.
Fact: Lupus does involve the immune system but its cause is unknown. HIV causes AIDS.

Myth: Lupus is a form of cancer.
Fact: Lupus is an autoimmune disease.

Myth: Lupus is contagious.
Fact: Again, the cause is unknown but you definitely can't catch it.

201

> Myth: Only black women get lupus.
> *Fact: Black men and other people of color also get lupus, but at lower rates than black women.*

What Causes Lupus?

Again, no one knows the cause of lupus. But because the disease tends to run in families, some experts suspect that people inherit the tendency to develop lupus, which is then triggered or made active by some internal or external factors such as hormones or toxins in the environment. An Emory University study published in 1997 found that African-Americans in a North Georgia community that had a history of long-term exposure to industrial emissions also had a significantly high rate of lupus. Though not a case of cause and effect, the study suggests that exposure to pollution can increase the risk of lupus.

Many Faces of Lupus

Lupus is a complex disease that affects different women differently. Sometimes called "the great imitator" or "masquerador," lupus has different forms and a range of symptoms. It is also difficult to diagnose because it resembles other conditions and there is no one "lupus test." Becoming an expert on the disease will help make it less daunting and easier to manage.

Forms of Lupus

Typically when people talk about lupus, they are referring to systemic lupus erythematosus. That is the most common form of the disease, but there are three types of lupus.

Systemic lupus erythematosus, or SLE, is an autoimmune condition in which the immune system produces an abundance of antibodies—blood proteins that normally protect us from harm—that attack healthy tissues in the body as if they were foreign invaders.

These destructive antibodies are known as autoantibodies. By attacking the body's cells and tissues, autoantibodies cause inflammation and pain in one or more areas of the body, which may include the skin, joints, kidneys, lung, heart, and brain. If the disease is not treated and damage to organs goes unchecked, SLE can be fatal.

Discoid lupus erythematosus, or DLE, is a form of the condition that mainly affects the skin. People with DLE usually have a red, raised rash on the face or other parts of the body. About one in ten people with DLE will develop SLE.

Drug-induced lupus, which is similar to SLE, is typically a temporary condition triggered by long-term use of certain medications. According to the Lupus Foundation of America, these drugs include Procainamide (Procan, Pronestyl), for irregular heart rhythm abnormalities; Hydralazine (Apresoline, Apresazide), for high blood pressure; Isoniazid (INH) for tuberculosis; Quinidine, for irregular heart rhythm; and Phenytoin (Dilantin), for seizures. When a patient stops taking the medication, the disease goes away within a matter of several days or several months.

Signs and Symptoms

Lupus got its name from its most prominent symptom—a telltale red rash on the face that resembles, some believe, the bite of a wolf. The rash may also take the shape of a butterfly spread across the nose and cheeks. Not every women with lupus will have the same symptoms. Common ones include:

- Red rash on face or other body parts
- Painful or swollen joints
- Unexplained fever
- Chest pain with breathing
- Unusual loss of hair
- Pale or purple fingers or toes from cold or stress
- Sensitivity to the sun
- Nausea and/or vomiting
- Abdominal pain

- Low white blood cell or platelet count
- Mouth sores
- Headache
- Swollen glands
- Extreme fatigue
- Unusual weight gain or loss

Women might also experience convulsions, hallucinations, and a greater susceptibility to common infections, bone fractures, kidney disease, and heart disease. A study recently conducted by the University of Pittsburgh concluded that women ages 35 to 44 with lupus were several times more likely to have a heart attack than women without lupus. The lupus subjects who had heart disease had it at an earlier age than those without the disease.

Because lupus is sometimes active and sometimes in remission, symptoms may arise or flare up unexpectedly. These active periods or "flares" may occur in response to triggers such as stress, sunlight, viral infections, and particular foods and medications, such as estrogen replacement therapy. Some women with lupus suffer more during pregnancy and shortly after (see "Lupus and Pregnancy").

Diagnosis

To diagnose lupus, a health care provider will take note of your medical history and symptoms. In addition to testing your blood count, blood chemistries, and urine, your provider may run a number of laboratory tests to determine whether lupus is present. These include:

- Erythrocyte sedimentation rate (ESR): a blood test that checks for inflammation in the body.
- Antinuclear antibody test (ANA): a test for the presence of antibodies that attack inside the nucleus of cells.
- Additional autoantibody tests: with names like anti-Sm, anti-RNP, anti-Ro and anti-La, these tests all reveal the presence of antibodies that react against a patient's own tissue.

- Serum complement level: a test that reveals the level of blood proteins known as complements. They are often low in people with lupus.
- Syphilis test: this common test may be positive in people with lupus, even if they don't actually have syphilis.

Your practitioner may also perform a skin or kidney biopsy to confirm the diagnosis. Because there is no one test for lupus, it may take months or even years to detect.

Living with Lupus

Because lupus has no cure, living with it means first and foremost listening to your body. Know what your symptoms are and identify those factors—stress, certain foods, sunlight—that worsen symptoms for you. Then, do what you must do to minimize the triggers. When flare-ups occur, take care of yourself—slow down and seek medical care when necessary.

Treatment

Because of the potentially serious nature of this disease, women with lupus must be under the regular care of a general practitioner or specialist such as a rheumatologist, a medical doctor specializing in diseases of the joints, bones, and muscles. Depending on the severity of your condition, you may need to see one provider or a team of providers. Don't just seek care when you feel bad; regular checkups can help minimize flare-ups of lupus and prevent serious complications. Be sure to tell your provider if you experience new symptoms or if side effects to treatment are bothersome. To maintain your overall health, continue to get your eye, dental, and gynecological exams routinely.

The standard medical treatment for lupus is corticosteroids, hormonal medications that reduce inflammation. Because corticosteroids such as prednisone are powerful drugs that can cause undesirable side effects, your provider should prescribe the lowest dose you need to ease symptoms. To lessen inflammation, lupus patients may also take over-the-counter NSAIDS, or nonsteroidal anti-inflammatory drugs such as Advil or Aleve. Though these medications keep people with lupus comfortable, they produce side effects. Because long-term corticosteroid use weakens bones, women with lupus are five times more likely to have fractures which threaten their overall health., according to a recent Northwestern University study.

Natural Complementary Solutions

In addition to your medical treatment, several preventive and alternative strategies will keep you strong and keep symptoms at bay.

Lifestyle. Keep up a regular exercise regimen to preserve strength and energy. Good workouts for women with lupus include walking, swimming, or biking according to the Lupus Foundation of America. Weight-bearing routines such as walking will help keep bones, which can be weakened by corticosteroid treatment, strong. Get sufficient rest. Stay out of the sun or guard yourself with hats, sun-protective clothing, and sunscreen.

Nutrition. Take note of foods that may be trigger flare-ups and avoid them entirely. Eat balanced meals with plenty of fresh vegetables and fruits. Eating omega-3 fatty-acid-rich fish such as salmon and mackerel may help alleviate joint pain and inflammation.

Supplements/Herbs. In addition to a multivitamin-mineral supplement, talk to your provider about taking calcium and vitamin D if you are on corticosteroid treatment, which can weaken bones.

Mind-Body Methods. Relaxation is key to preventing stress-related flare-ups. You might practice deep breathing or meditation once or twice a day to calm yourself. Or perhaps a relaxing hobby such as knitting, crafts, or cooking will keep your mind off stressful thoughts. Yoga may be especially beneficial for relaxation and release of tension. To keep your spirits up, join or create a support group (see the Resources), or talk to a mental health professional. Call on friends, family, and neighbors when you need help with the tasks of daily living or emotional support.

Hands-On Healing. Massage may relieve both physical tension and discomfort—and simply make you feel good. Acupuncture may also alleviate pain.

Lupus and Pregnancy

Years ago, doctors told women with lupus not to get pregnant because pregnancy was too risky for them and their unborn child. That's no longer true. Most women with lupus can have safe pregnancies even though they're considered high-risk. To increase your odds for a healthy pregnancy and delivery of a normal, healthy baby, follow these important tips:

- Plan to conceive when your lupus is under good control or in remission. Getting pregnant while your lupus is active may result in a miscarriage, a stillbirth, or a serious complication.
- Choose an obstetrician with experience managing high-risk pregnancies and who is associated with a hospital specializing in high-risk deliveries.
- Eat a well-balanced diet. Avoid excessive weight gain, smoking, and alcohol.
- Take prescribed medications as directed, but never take any medicines—over-the-counter drugs, herbs, or vitamins—without your doctor's okay.
- Report all signs of potential flares (headaches, abdominal pain, swelling) to your doctor immediately.
- Rest and de-stress your life as much as possible.

Emotional Impact of the Disease

Having any chronic disease can be frightening and emotionally draining. And because lupus is poorly understood and unpredictable, it can be particularly unsettling. The physical symptoms are just one aspect of the challenge of coping with lupus. You may also have to take many sick days or disability, and struggle to get insurance coverage and pay for treatment. Loved ones and friends may not always understand what you're going through or be there for you in a way that you need. Because of these difficulties, many women with lupus suffer depression, particularly during or after a bout of disease or a hospitalization.

Caring for your emotions and spirit is as key to your well-being as any physical treatment.

Learn as much as you can about lupus. Knowledge is power. Don't simply rely on your physician's knowledge; collect and absorb as much information as you can find about your illness. Check out books on lupus at your library or bookstore; contact lupus organizations (see the Resources) to request information or browse websites; read newspaper and magazine articles. Replace fear with information.

Take an active role in your healing. Again, don't rely on your doctor or treatment to keep you well. Exercise, eat a nutritious natural diet, and get plenty of rest. Slow down and take extra special care of yourself during a flare-up.

Become a lupus activist. Fuel any frustrations your have about having lupus into fighting it for yourself and others. Join or create a support group. Contact lupus organizations (see the Resources) for information on how to participate in lupus research and advocacy.

Maintain a positive outlook. Though lupus is serious, these days the majority of people with lupus who receive good treatment can expect to live as long as people without lupus. That is excellent news. Focusing on the positive aspects of your life will greatly increase your mind-body's ability to manage the condition. Do what makes you happy—spend time with family or friends; indulge in a favorite hobby—every day, and surround yourself with supportive, positive people.

Resources

American Lupus Society, 3914 Del Amo Boulevard, Suite 922, Torrance, CA 90503; (800) 331-1802.

Lupus Foundation of America (LFA), Inc., 1300 Piccard Drive, Suite 200, Rockville, MD 20850; (301) 670-9292, (800) 558-0121; http://www.lupus.org/lupus

The Lupus Handbook for Women, by Robin Dibner, MD, and Carol Colman (Fireside).

National Arthritis and Musculoskeletal and Skin Diseases Institute, Box AMS, 900 Rockville Pike, Bethesda, MD 20892.

Chapter 12

~

Confronting Cancer

NATURAL WOMAN: DONNA GREEN-GOODMAN

In July 1996, Donna Green-Goodman heard the words so many women fear: You have breast cancer. Not only did she have a serious disease at age 37, but it was an aggressive form of cancer. Her doctors did not believe she would survive more than two to five years, even with the most advanced treatment. "I couldn't believe it," recalls the Atlanta-based health educator. "How could this happen? I had always been a healthy person." But despite her initial panic, Donna took control. She agreed to having the tumor removed through a surgical procedure called lumpectomy. But instead of going through with radiation, chemotherapy, and a stem-cell transplant to destroy any remaining cancer cells that might still be in her body, Donna chose a more natural approach to complete her healing. "I asked, 'What happens to the women who do these treatments?'" Donna says. "They said 70 percent of women with my type of cancer die. I asked 'Well, what guarantee can you give me?' 'There is no guarantee,' they said. 'You're telling me there's no guarantee and people who do what you say die? I need to find something else.'"

She heard about a nearby health facility, Wildwood Lifestyle Center and Hospital in Wildwood, Georgia, which offered a program focusing on good nutrition, exercise, and other noninvasive methods. After registering with the facility's ten-day program, Donna adopted a strict vegetarian diet, including lots of carrot juice and vegetable juices. She was also treated with a form of hydrotherapy that stimulates the immune system by immersing a patient in warm water to raise the body temperature and trigger white blood cells. Walking outdoors for exercise and massage completed her therapy.

After leaving the lifestyle program, Donna returned to her original doctor. She decided to go ahead with radiation treatment, but after four weeks, she'd had enough of the nausea, fatigue, and burning sensations in her breast. She returned home, continuing the habits she'd learned at Wildwood. Within months, tests and blood work indicated that she was free of the cancer.

Despite the initial predictions, Donna is still going strong four years later. She maintains her diet, walks every day, and gets massages and hydrotherapy a few times a year. Since her healing, Donna has hooked up with other health professionals in order to create a health program, Lifestyle Principles, Inc., in Decatur, which offers the same type of services she received at Wildwood to others on an outpatient basis. She's also written a book about her experience called Somethin' to Shout About: Celebrating Health and Healing Through Diet and Lifestyles. *Saying good-bye to the superwoman, she's put stress in perspective. "You look at life differently," she notes. "It's not about my breast, it's about my whole life being more in balance and healthy. If I'm not healthy, what's my point in being here?"*

Cancer is not one disease but many. In the black community, we hear a lot about cancers of the breast and prostate but the term "cancer" refers to more than 100 conditions affecting nearly every part of the body. Cancer occurs when normal cells grow unchecked, forming tumors and sometimes spreading to other tissues and organs. Health experts don't fully understand what causes cancer but many suspect that a combination of genetic, environmental, and lifestyle factors contributes to the illness.

Cancer is a common disease, but it is an especially prevalent problem in the black community. According to the American Cancer Society's *Cancer Facts & Figures for African Americans, 1998-1999,* Blacks have a higher incidence of several forms of cancer, including colon and rectal cancer, lung cancer, and cancer of the prostate, than any other racial or ethnic group in the United States. We are also more likely to die of these cancers and of breast cancer. Experts attribute this bad news to many issues, including poverty, lack of awareness, inadequate access to health care, among others. Late detection—and late treatment—is a key factor that makes us especially vulnerable to malignancies of all kinds.

Talking about cancer is not as taboo now as it was in the past. Referring to cancer as the "Big C" or "C-A" has reflected our fear of even uttering the word we associate with suffering and death. Cancer is a very serious disease but it is much more survivable today than it once was. Talking about cancer will help us prevent it. And the use of natural therapies that complement conventional cancer treatments will improve our chances of overcoming it.

Leading Cancer Sites in Black Women

Breast
Lung and bronchus
Colon and rectum
Uterine corpus
Uterine cervix
Ovary
Pancreas
Non-Hodgkin's lymphoma
Kidney
Multiple myeloma

Source: *Cancer Facts & Figures for African Americans*, 1998–1999, American Cancer Society.

Cancer's Causes

Many different factors contribute to the development of cancer but the exact cause is still a mystery. Most folks are surprised to learn that our bodies produce cancer cells along with the billions of other cells they produce every day. Because of genetic defects or exposure to carcinogens such as tobacco smoke or sunlight, these cells reproduce uncontrollably. When the body is healthy, the immune system quickly identifies and destroys cancer cells. But when the body is not at its strongest, cancer cells can take root and multiply. To prevent cancer or to completely heal from it, the immune system and body must be kept strong through a natural anticancer lifestyle. This includes avoiding those factors within our control that weaken our natural defenses and put us at risk.

What could raise your risk of cancer? The following internal and external factors:

Age. Your chance of getting any form of a cancer increases as you age. This may be because of increased or prolonged exposure to carcinogens as well as because our immune systems weaken as we get older.

Smoking. Tobacco smoke is the most important factor in the development of lung cancer, the leading cause of cancer deaths in black women. (Radon gas also contributes to a minority of lung cancers.) Smoking also increases the risk of cancers of the mouth, larynx and bladder. Studies tell us that even exposure to secondhand smoke is hazardous.

Poor, Unnatural Diet. As much as one-third of all cancer deaths may be associated with diet, say experts at the American Cancer Society. The foods we eat can improve, or hinder, our body's ability to stave off cancer. For example, scientists have discovered that a variety of chemicals found in fresh vegetables and fruits actually protect our cells from invasion by carcinogens or block cancer cell growth. Conversely, diets low in plant foods and high in fat leave our bodies vulnerable to cancer.

Inactivity. Studies suggest that people who don't exercise routinely have a greater chance of getting cancer than those who are fit. This may be because physical activity helps prevent weight gain (obesity is associated with cancer), strengthen the immune system, and balance our hormones including estrogen, which may promote the growth of hormone-related cancers such as breast cancer.

Overweight. Excess body fat may increase the risk of breast cancer because fat produces estrogen.

Radiation and Environmental Chemicals. Radiation from X rays, the sun, and nuclear waste raises the risk of cancer. Exposure to other toxins such as asbestos raises lung cancer risk.

Heredity. Certain cancers appear to run in families. In some of those cases, specific genes may be partly responsible for the development of the disease. If cancer is common in your family, especially among close relatives such as a parent or sibling, your chance of getting cancer increases.

Viruses. The presence of certain viruses in the body may lead to harmful cell changes. Hepatitis B virus can cause liver cancer. The human papillomavirus is present in most (if not all) cervical cancer cases.

Alcohol. Drinking too much alcohol raises estrogen levels, which may explain the link between alcohol and breast cancer risk in women. It may also contribute to other cancers.

Sun Exposure. Though blacks have natural skin protection with melanin, some of us do get skin cancer. The American Cancer Society estimates there were 100 new cases of melanoma among black women in 1999. Radiation from the sun's ultraviolet rays is the culprit.

Preventing Cancer

Although there are no guarantees that we can prevent cancer, we can greatly diminish the risk of developing the disease through natural means. The fact that experts consider smoking and diet to be responsible for two-thirds of all cancer deaths tells us that healthy behavior is the most important cancer prevention aid we have. Our bodies need to be strong on mental, physical, emotional, and spiritual levels in order to stop cancer cells from forming and growing in the first place. No one strategy will prevent cancer definitively, but a mind-body-spirit approach is our best defense.

Lifestyle. Exercise four to five times per week for thirty minutes or longer. This routine physical activity reduces stress and the risk of hormone-related cancers such as breast cancer. Exercise decreases the amount of circulating estrogen, a factor in breast cancer. It also helps us maintain a healthy weight. Anything you like to do consistently—walking, African dance, water fitness classes—will do.

Nutrition. Eat a natural diet that emphasizes vegetables, fruits, and whole grains. *Colorful fresh vegetables*—dark greens and red, orange, and yellow vegetables—contain the most potent cancer-fighting pigments. Produce to add to your shopping list: collards, kale, broccoli, turnip greens, carrots, red peppers, dark leafy greens, tomatoes, citrus fruits, grapes, and strawberries. Make sure to eat one or two servings of such fresh produce at every meal. Do not overcook vegetables but steam them or eat them raw for the greatest benefit. In addition, whole grains and beans provide the *fiber* our bodies need to fend off colon cancer. *Soy* foods may also protect against hormone-related cancers such as breast cancer.

Foods to avoid: high-fat meats and dairy products; cured or smoked meats; sugar; alcohol.

Supplements. In addition to a multivitamin-mineral supplement, antioxidant vitamins and mineral supplements may help the body stop free radicals from damaging cells. These include vitamins A, C, and E and selenium.

Herbs. Garlic tablets may help in blocking cancer cell growth and boosting immunity.

Mind-Body Methods. Practice a relaxation technique (deep breathing, meditation, prayer) that you enjoy daily to prevent stress from weakening your immune system or leading you to unhealthy behaviors. If stress and anxiety are overwhelming, talk to a therapist or join a support group.

Hands-On Healing. Regular massage or reflexology treatments can help you completely relax and ease stress.

Early Detection Methods

If cancer does occur in your body, detecting it at an early stage greatly increases your chance of survival. Some women avoid tests out of fear of learning the worst. But if you don't even know you have a disease, your chance of overcoming it diminishes dramatically. Between 1990 and 1995, black women diagnosed with localized breast cancer—cancer contained in the breast—had a five-year survival rate of 89 percent, according to the American Cancer Society. That rate dropped to 14 percent for sisters diagnosed with breast cancer that had spread to distant areas of the body.

A growing number of tests help you and your doctors locate abnormal cells or tumors as soon as they are detectable. Understanding each of the tests—and when you should have them—will help you get a step ahead of cancer. They include:

Breast Self-Exam (BSE)

When to do it: every month beginning at age 18. If you are premenopausal, the best time of the month to perform a breast self-exam is a few days after your period when hormone-related changes that may make breasts lumpier subside. The self-exam includes three parts:

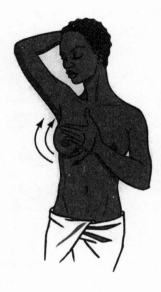

Breast Self-Exam
Get in the habit of checking your breasts every month. The best time to perform a self-exam (see description) is a few days after your period.

1. While lying down with your left arm raised above your head, use the flattened fingers of your right hand to examine the left breast. Beginning with the nipple area and working outward in a circular (or up and down) pattern, press into the breast tissue to feel for lumps. Do this slowly and attentively. Don't forget to feel your armpit as well. Also squeeze the nipple for signs of discharge. Then repeat on the other breast.
2. Standing in front of a mirror, firmly place your hands on your hips. Then raise your hands overhead. Look for any dimpling in the skin or asymmetry in breast shape, size, or color.
3. In the shower or sitting up in a bath, repeat Step 1. Use soapy hands to glide over wet skin. The moisture and change in position may make it easier to detect lumps.

Many women forget to examine their breasts or are simply afraid to do it. However, most breast lumps are found by women or their partners. You are your first line of defense against breast cancer. It is important to become familiar with the way your breasts feel so that if a lump occurs—and most are benign—you can detect it and see your doctor right away. If you are not sure how to perform the self-exam, talk to your ob-gyn. See the Resources for organizations that provide materials on BSE.

Clinical Breast Exam (CBE)

When to do it: every year beginning at age 18. A clinical breast exam is simply a manual exam much like BSE that your doctor or a nurse performs in the doctor's office. It should be part of your annual ob-gyn examination. If you or your mate should discover a lump at home, see your provider for a clinical exam.

Mammogram

When to do it: Once at age 35 then annually after age 40. To perform this X ray of the breast, a radiologist or qualified technician will place each breast between plates that compress them mildly in order to get the best picture. Two X rays of each breast are taken. Getting a mammogram may be uncomfortable, but the test takes only about fifteen minutes. Your radiologist or technician will then read the X ray and give you results in the same visit.

Some women are concerned about the radiation emitted during a mammogram. A small dose is absorbed by the body but the benefit probably outweighs the risk. Mammograms can detect small lumps up to two years before they can be felt by hand.

Before you schedule your first mammogram, ask the radiologist or technician whether her/his facility uses up-to-date technology and complies with federal regulations. Mammogram technology continues to improve. For example, digital mammograms generate computerized images of the breast that a technician can alter in order to see abnormalities. However, digital mammography is not available nationwide and does not replace traditional mammography.

Sonogram

The same technology used to determine the size and sex of a developing fetus may be used in addition to mammography to detect breast lumps. Also known as a sonogram, ultrasound may be particularly effective with young women, who tend to have denser breast tissue than older women.

Pelvic Exam

When to do it: every year for women age 18 and older. The purpose of this important exam is to check the vulva, vagina, fallopian tubes, ovaries, and uterus for any signs of infection, growths, or other abnormalities. During this exam, which usually takes no more than 15 to 20 minutes, you lie down on your back with knees bent and feet in stirrups. Your ob-gyn should first open your vaginal lips and examine the vulva with gloved hands. Then by inserting a speculum to widen the walls of the vagina, your ob-gyn will take a look at the walls of your vagina and cervix. With the speculum in place, your ob-gyn will perform a Pap test (see below). Lastly, after removing the speculum, the doctor will place two fingers of one hand in the vagina while pressing down on your abdomen. This allows her/him to feel your pelvic organs and detect such problems as fibroid tumors and ovarian cysts. To complete the exam, your doctor will quickly insert a finger in your rectum to check for growths.

Pelvic exams may be uncomfortable, especially for women with a history of sexual abuse. To make the exam more comfortable for you, you may want to ask for a female doctor or a nurse to be present while a male doctor performs the procedures. Also, before the exam starts, don't be afraid to ask for socks to be placed on your feet to prevent them from getting cold or for the speculum to be warmed. In order to relax during the exam, concentrate on breathing fully.

Pap Test

When to do it: every year for women age 18 and older. Also known as the Pap smear, this exam's purpose is to check cervical cells for abnormal changes that could potentially lead to cervical cancer. (The Pap test can also detect common sexually transmitted infections.) To perform the test, your ob-gyn inserts a speculum to open the vaginal walls followed by a long cotton swab that is used to swab cervical cells for testing. The cells are smeared on a glass slide, which is then sent to a laboratory where they are examined under a microscope for changes. In most cases, cervical cell changes are self-limiting and do no indicate cancer. When in doubt, an ob-gyn might want to perform a biopsy to remove more cells to get a closer look. Pap test technology has also improved in recent years. A relatively new test called Thin Prep allows your doctor to preserve cells in liquid before they are examined, which improves the chance of detecting abnormalities. Since it was introduced the late 1940s, the Pap test has substantially reduced the death rate from cervical cancer.

Having the Pap test done annually during your childbearing years (and as often as your ob-gyn recommends thereafter) is critical. Black women have three times the cervical cancer rate of white women, and we are twice as likely to die of the disease because of late diagnosis. Cervical cancer does not cause symptoms until it is advanced.

Colorectal Screening

When to do it: every year after age 40. Colon cancer screening includes at least one of three test: a digital rectal exam, fecal occult blood test, and proctoscopy. Though screening rates have increased among blacks, we still have a lower five-year survival rate than whites.

Skin Self-Exam

A self-check for new moles or other skin lesions can help you detect skin cancer early. Remove clothes and examine your skin in front of a full-length mirror in a well-lit room. Use a hand mirror to view the back of your body. In addition to checking for moles, check for any sores that haven't healed in three weeks. If an existing mole changes in shape, size, or color, see your physician.

Biopsies

When any form of cancer is suspected, your doctor may remove tissue to get a closer look at it under a microscope. Depending on the form of cancer, a biopsy may take a few minutes or longer to perform. Your doctor may give you your results within the same day or week.

Too Young for Breast Cancer?

The incidence of breast cancer is low in younger women, but for unknown reasons, it has risen among black women under age 45. Worse, for younger sisters, the disease is often more aggressive and it can be deadlier because we often detect it at a late stage. Cancer studies have found that mortality rates can be reduced dramatically through early detection and timely treatment. To protect yourself, regardless of age, get to know your breasts through monthly self-exams. Get yearly clinical breast exams at your ob-gyn's office. If you find a lump or have unexplained breast pains, ask your doctor for a mammogram (coupled with a sonogram if you're under age 40). Don't let anyone tell you "you're too young," especially if the disease runs in your family. If a suspicious lump or mass is found, be sure to get follow-up tests. If you disagree with your doctor's assessment, get a second opinion.

NATURAL WOMAN: CYNTHIA PITRE

Cynthia Pitre first thought she had pulled a muscle when she noticed a sensation between her left armpit and breast. But when the area hardened into a lump, she went to the doctor. A mammogram and biopsy later, Cynthia learned she had breast cancer at age 38.

A lumpectomy to remove the tumor was only partly successful: Tests showed cancerous tissue remained in her breast and was spreading. Doctor after doctor told her to have more surgery and either undergo chemotherapy or radiation. Frustrated with her choices, she finally decided to explore alternatives to conventional cancer treatment. First, Cynthia returned to healers who practiced a type of talk therapy called Sunan where she was able to completely release some painful memories from her past and heal on a deeply spiritual level. Then, upon the advice of an alternative practitioner, she switched to a largely raw vegetable and fruit diet, which also consisted of nuts and seeds. Colonic hydrotherapy treatments completed her regimen. A year after her diagnosis, a mammogram revealed only calcifications—white specks of tissue—in her breast, but no cancer. Three years later, in 1998, Pitre's mammograms still showed she was cancer free.

Cynthia continues with her vegetarian diet and colon therapy, which she now administers to others. She also gets on the treadmill or a stationary bicycle four to five days a week in addition to lifting light weights. Weekly Swedish massages for relaxation and biweekly lymphatic massages add to her health routine. Most critically, Cynthia persists in putting her health first. "I [am] not going to make company business more important than my health—that was a decision I made long ago when I started healing myself," she says. The focus on health from the beginning of her day until the end is key. "How many people wake up and say what am I going to do with my health? How am I going to lower my stress and nurture myself today?" As a cancer survivor and the owner of Years to Your Life, her own colonic therapy business, Cynthia knows of what she speaks and shares this wisdom daily with clients.

Complementary Care

Because cancer is serious and life-threatening, the best approach to healing is to first learn everything you can about the condition and avail yourself of the very best treatment options—conventional and alternative. Especially in advanced stages of cancer, hope and prayer alone will not cure the disease. But natural healing strategies can strengthen the body and help prevent further cancer growth while modern medical techniques stop the disease by removing or destroying malignant tumors or cells.

Complementary cancer care includes any natural remedy that strengthens the body during conventional cancer treatment or that alleviates the side effects of such treatment. Conventional cancer treatment involves one or more of the following: *surgery* to remove tumors and any cancerous tissue; *chemotherapy* or the use of powerful chemicals to destroy cancer cells; *radiation* or the use of X rays to destroy cancer cells; or *immunotherapy* to boost the immune system in order to fight cancer. Bone marrow transplants and cancer prevention drugs like tamoxifen are newer medical approaches. The first three—surgery, chemo, and radiation—may be very effective in stopping cancer but also often harm healthy tissue and cause troublesome side effects such as pain, nausea, fatigue, weight loss or gain, hair loss, etc. They also do not address the whole body and all the factors that contribute to cancer or its recurrence. That is why complementary care may not only make conventional cancer treatment easier to bear but also more effective because the body is healing in more ways than one.

Before deciding on any particular complementary or alternative therapy, you should do your own research and ask lots of questions. Go to the library and bookstore and read any books, magazine articles, and studies you can get your hands on. Also talk to others who have cancer or who have survived it using complementary care. But understand that what works for one person may not work for you. Carefully consider the effort and cost involved in any therapy. Gather information and make the decision that is best for you.

Complementary cancer therapies generally work to either detoxify the body—or rid it of harmful substances from food, our environment, or cancer treatment itself—and/or strengthen the immune system to enable the body to fight cancer. No single therapy is a cure-all but part of a program to restore health.

Whatever approach or approaches you choose, be certain to discuss them with your medical doctors as well as your alternative medicine practitioners. Not all therapies are compatible. If a doctor does not support your decision to use alternatives, consider seeking another physician more sensitive to your needs. Having sympathetic caregivers will help as you experiment with a therapy or therapies and evaluate your progress.

Lifestyle. Exercise improves immune system function and prevents hormone imbalance. Low-impact activities such as qigong may work best for those undergoing treatment.

Nutrition. Eat a balanced natural diet high in cancer-fighting vegetables and fruits. Cruciferous vegetables such as broccoli, kale, and collard greens contain powerful cancer-fighting substances. Soy products, garlic, and green tea also naturally help the body stop cancer. Nutritional therapies may include vegetarianism, a raw food diet, macrobiotics, juicing, or fasting. Avoid animal fat, salt, and sugar.

Supplements/Herbs. Intravenous vitamin and minerals; metabolic therapy, which includes the daily intake of vitamins, minerals and enzymes; and homeopathy.

Mind-Body Methods. Counseling; support groups; relaxation; spiritual support; hypnosis; visualization; journaling.

Hands-On Healing. Acupuncture/acupressure for pain and nausea associated with cancer treatment; lymphatic massage; colonic irrigation therapy; enemas; herbal wraps; hypothermia.

For a complete list of alternative cancer centers that provide therapies, from Ayurveda to ozone therapy, read *Third Opinion: An International Directory to Alternative Therapy Centers for the Treatment and Prevention of Cancer and Other Degenerative Diseases* by John M. Fink.

Resources

American Cancer Society, National Office, 1599 Clifton Road, NE, Atlanta, GA 30329; (800) ACS-2345.

National Alliance of Breast Cancer Organizations (NABCO), 1180 Avenue of the Americas, New York, NY 10036.

National Black Leadership Initiative on Cancer, National Cancer Institute, Executive Plaza N., Room 240, Bethesda, MD 20892.

National Cancer Institute Information Service, National Institutes of Health, Bethesda, MD 20205; (800) 4-Cancer.

Breast Cancer? Breath Health! The Wise Woman Way, by Susan S. Weed (Ash Tree Publishing).

What to Eat if You Have Cancer: A Guide to Adding Nutritional Therapy to Your Treatment Plan, by Maureen Keane, MS, and Daniella Chase, MS (Contemporary Books).

Women Confront Cancer: Making Medical History by Choosing Alternative and Complementary Therapies, by Margaret J. Wooddell and David J. Hess (New York University Press).

Traditional Chinese Medicine: A Woman's Guide to Healing from Breast Cancer, by Nan Lu, OMD, Lac, with Ellen Schaplowsky (Avon).

Third Opinion: An International Directory to Alternative Therapy Centers for the Treatment and Prevention of Cancer & Other Degenerative Diseases, by John M. Fink (Avery Publishing).

Chapter 13

~

Coping with Chronic Conditions: Hypertension, Diabetes, Heart Disease

NATURAL WOMAN: ANGELL JACOBS

In addition to inheriting family traits such as eye color and hair texture, Angell Jacobs inherited her relatives' tendency to have high blood pressure. Diagnosed with the condition in her twenties, Angell initially took hypertension medication to keep her pressure down. But after a few years, she decided to seek an alternative to the drugs she didn't want to have to take all her life. A friend recommended a naturopathic physician, Dr. Andrea Sullivan of Washington D.C. who helped Angell gradually shift to a more natural lifestyle. The prescription consisted first of a significant change in diet—lots of vegetables, fruit, and fish, and fewer processed foods and meat. Angell also started taking pressure-lowering herbs such as garlic daily. A series of colon hydrotherapy treatments added to the regimen. Within just a few months of following the naturopath's advice, Angell lost 13 pounds and her pressure had lowered even more than with the medications alone.

Her last healing step was to add exercise in the form of power walking for a half hour a day, three days a week. This gave Angell

227

energy and helped her relieve the stress of her job as a management consultant. After sticking to her natural diet, herbs, and exercise for two years, Angell talked to her physician about ceasing the pressure-lowering drugs. Several months after doing so, her pressure was still a normal 110/70. Today Angell fully embraces her new lifestyle. "It's really empowered me to take care of myself and live the most healthful life that I could," she says.

In many black families, we commonly talk about relatives who "have sugar" or someone whose "pressure is up." In fact, diabetes and hypertension are so widespread, they seem almost inevitable, especially among black women. One in four black women over age 55 has type II diabetes. Sisters are twice as likely as a white woman to have high blood pressure. These conditions are examples of the major threat to black women's survival today—chronic diseases. Heart disease, stroke, and most recently HIV/AIDS also top the list of these long-term health challenges. (Though AIDS is caused by infection, with adequate treatment, it can become a lifelong or chronic disease.)

Black women are especially at risk for developing or dying from chronic diseases for a variety of reasons including poverty, racism, and even genetics. But all of these conditions are preventable, and to a certain extent, treatable, through natural means. Even if we are predisposed to, say, high blood pressure because many of our relatives have the disease, we can still lower our risk of getting it. And those of us who already suffer from diabetes, for example, can either manage it or at least minimize the need for insulin or other diabetes medications by eating a natural, wholesome diet and becoming more physically active. Though drug treatment may be necessary to control certain chronic diseases, natural lifestyle choices and remedies can lessen our dependence on medications and strengthen the body, mind, and spirit in spite of illness.

Preventing or controlling a chronic condition requires first and foremost self-care. Whether we use natural remedies, medications, or both, we must make the care of our own bodies as urgent a priority as the jobs, families, and other responsibilities that we give our time and attention to every day. Caring for ourselves is a lifelong, or chronic, challenge for all black women but especially so if you are living with a major illness. Self-care—eating well, exercising, easing stress, and taking medication when necessary—is the key to our survival.

Natural Healing and Our History

The chronic conditions many African-Americans are prone to today were not common among our African ancestors or even contemporary Africans. Coronary heart disease, the leading cause of death for all Americans, was rare worldwide before 1900 but is still almost unheard of throughout sub-Saharan Africa today. Hypertension was also uncommon and remains rare among rural Africans though it is present among those living in cities, who tend to consume more salt. The difference between rural and urban Africans mirrors somewhat the difference between our ancestors and ourselves: Indigenous Africans tend to eat a low-salt, low saturated-fat diet, and they exert themselves physically through the chores of daily living, burning any excess calories and sweating out any excess salt. We tend to eat high animal fat or processed foods flavored with too much salt or sugar while getting little physical activity and carrying excess weight to boot. It is these lifestyle factors—not our race or ethnic background—that make for our high incidence of chronic diseases.

Some health experts believe blacks inherited a tendency to retain salt because those Africans who were able to retain more salt and fluids in the arid climate in Africa or under the harsh conditions of the slave trade were the ones to survive and pass on their genes. But only three out of four black people with high blood pressure are "salt-sensitive," and the trait alone does not make us hypertensive. The trait combined with a high-salt, low-potassium American diet, among other negative lifestyle forces, is what gives rise to the high blood pressure problem in our community today.

Chronic Conditions

The following are among the leading causes of death and disability in black women. Here's what you need to know about them:

Hypertension or High Blood Pressure

What It Is

The "pressure" in high blood pressure refers to the force of blood pumping through our arteries. This pressure normally increases each time we exercise or experience stress. But if that force or pressure remains high even when we are at rest, we have high blood pressure or hypertension. The condition may be caused by many factors including our genetic makeup; a high-fat, high-salt diet; excess weight; smoking; and excessive drinking. Ongoing stress, including the stress of racism, may also contribute to hypertension. High blood pressure does not typically cause symptoms until it is quite serious. However, it is often called a silent killer because, unchecked, hypertension puts us in danger of developing heart attacks and strokes. There is no cure, but hypertension can be controlled.

While checking your blood pressure, a doctor measures both the force of blood while the heart is pumping (systolic) and while at rest (diastolic). Normal blood pressure is 120/80. The following blood pressure categories will help you and your health care provider decide what type of treatment you need. (These categories are for people over age 18 who are not on antihypertensive medication.)

To be on the safe side, you should have your blood pressure checked every year by your health care provider or physician. If you have high-normal blood pressure or full-fledged hypertension, ask your doctor how often you should have your pressure checked—and stick to the schedule. You should also learn to check your own blood pressure at home so that you know where you are in terms of blood pressure control.

How to Detect It

	Systolic		Diastolic
Optimal	Less than 120		Less than 80
Normal	Less than 130	and	Less than 85
High normal	130–139	or	85–89
Hypertension			
Stage 1 (mild)	140–159	or	90–99
Stage 2 (moderate)	160–179	or	100–109
Stage 3 (severe)	180–209	or	110–119
Stage 4 (extremely severe*)	210 or higher	or	120 or higher

* requires immediate medical assistance

Prevention and Complementary Care

Lifestyle. Regular exercise helps to strengthen the heart and lower your resting heart rate. Briskly walk, take an exercise class, or play a sport four to five days per week.

Nutrition. A balanced, natural diet that is low in fat and sodium and high in potassium and other key nutrients is essential for stabilizing blood pressure. To minimize your salt intake, read food labels, avoid prepared foods and canned products, ask about salt content while eating out, and do not add salt while cooking or before eating a meal. See "The Diet That Stops Hypertension" for specific dietary recommendations.

Supplements/Herbs. A multivitamin-mineral supplement containing calcium, magnesium, potassium, and fiber might help. Garlic also works to lower blood pressure quite effectively.

Mind-Body Methods. Relaxation techniques will help you control stress. A form of meditation known as Transcendental Meditation has enabled blacks in studies to lower their blood pressure without medication. Another proven pressure-lowering technique is tai chi. Support groups and other social ties can help buffer the stress of racism—an underestimated factor in hypertension.

Hands-On Healing. Regular massages or foot reflexology treatments can counter the effects of stress.

The Diet that Stops Hypertension

Experts at the National Institutes of Health recently proved that specific changes in diet can lower blood pressure as effectively as medication. A clinical trial, which included many African-Americans, demonstrated that by consuming more vegetables and fruit and less fat, people at risk for hypertension, and those who already have a mild form of the condition, can lower their blood pressure—naturally—within weeks. Known as the DASH (Dietary Approaches to Stop Hypertension) diet, this eating plan may help prevent hypertension *and* lessen the need for medication in those with Stage 1 high blood pressure. The results occurred without any changes in salt intake, exercise, or alcohol consumption. Though not vegetarian, the diet is high in potassium, magnesium, calcium, and fiber. This is what it looks like, though for the full diet and sample menus, call 800-575-WELL or visit the National Heart Blood and Lung Institute website: http:nhlbi.nih.gov/nhlbi/nhlbi.htm.

Food Group	Daily Servings	Serving Sizes	Examples
Grains	7 to 8	1 slice bread; ½ cup dry cereal, cooked rice, or pasta	Whole wheat bread, grits, oatmeal
Vegetables	4 to 5	1 cup raw or ½ cup cooked vegetables, 6 ounces juice	Spinach, kale, tomatoes, peas, carrots, squash
Fruits	4 to 5	1 medium fruit, ¼ cup dried or ½ cup fresh or frozen fruit, 6 ounces juice	Orange, grapefruit, banana, raisins, prunes, grapes, melons

| | | | Table continued |
Food Group	Daily Servings	Serving Sizes	Examples
Low-fat dairy	2 to 3	8 ounces milk, 1 cup yogurt, 1.5 ounces cheese	Skim milk, low-fat yogurt, nonfat cheese
Fish, poultry, meat	2 to 3	3 ounces, cooked fish, poultry or meat	Lean cut; broiled or roasted; remove skin from poultry
Nuts, seeds, legumes	4 to 5 *per week*	1.5 ounces or ⅓ cup nuts, 1 ounce or 2 tablespoons seeds, 1 cup cooked legumes	Almonds, sunflower seeds, lentils, beans

Diabetes Type II

What It Is

It's been called "sugar" because diabetes results from the body's inability to produce or use insulin in order to convert sugar and other foods into energy. But it's more than a touch of sugar; diabetes is a quite serious and increasingly common disease. Most diabetics have type II or non-insulin-dependent diabetes mellitus, a condition caused by the body's inability to use insulin. (Type I diabetics, or those with insulin-dependent diabetes mellitus, produce little or no insulin.) Type II may be triggered by a combination of genetics; a high-fat, high-sugar diet; excess weight; lack of exercise; and excessive drinking. Half of all diabetics don't realize they have the disease because it does not cause obvious symptoms until it has caused complications. The signs include:

233

- Excessive thirst
- Excessive hunger
- Frequent urination
- Significant weight loss or gain
- Slow healing of bruises and cuts
- Frequent infections, including yeast infections and urinary tract infections
- Numbness or tingling in feet, hands, legs, or arms
- Blurred vision
- Fatigue

Untreated, diabetes can cause damage to nerves and blood vessels, raise the risk of hypertension and heart disease, and cause death. African-Americans are more likely to suffer adverse consequences of untreated or poorly treated diabetes, including blindness, limb amputations, and kidney failure. Diabetes type II is not curable but it can be controlled.

How to Detect It

Because a person can have type II diabetes for as many as ten years without knowing it, it is crucial to watch for the signs listed above. To catch diabetes before it causes damage, experts at the American Diabetes Association (ADA) recently changed the blood-sugar threshold that defines the disease. In the past, having a fasting blood sugar reading of 140 milligrams per deciliter meant you had diabetes. Today, the categories are as follows:

Normal	Less than 110 mg/dl
Impaired (at risk)	110 to 125 mg/dl
Diabetic	126 mg/dl or more

To determine your blood sugar level, the ADA recommends that all adults get tested beginning at age 45. Blacks and those with a family history of diabetes should be tested even earlier—as young as age 35 or younger. (See "Diabetes: Are You at Risk?") Pregnant women should also get tested around the sixth month because a form of diabetes known as gestational diabetes mellitus can develop while you are with child; it typically goes away after pregnancy but can cause complications. The testing usually involves a fasting blood glucose test, or a blood test taken after you have not eaten for about eight hours.

If you have higher than normal blood sugar levels—a condition known as impaired glucose tolerance—you may be able to make changes in your diet and exercise habits that will prevent or at least delay the onset of diabetes. However, if you have diabetes, you must be under the care of a physician. Lifestyle changes and weight loss can eliminate or at least reduce the need for insulin. Keeping a watchful eye on your blood sugar is key, so ask your doctor how often you should check it and how to check it at home.

Prevention and Complementary Care

Lifestyle. Talk to your health care provider about what a healthy weight is for you. Losing 10 pounds or more and keeping it off may make a difference. The best way to do this is through proper nutrition and consistent exercise. Frequent exercise can help stabilize blood sugar: One University of Pittsburgh study found that by exercising daily (walking, cycling) for one week, twelve overweight black women improved their insulin response significantly. Also see your eye doctor and dentist regularly to catch changes in vision and gum infections, which occur more often in diabetics.

Nutrition. Eating a balanced, natural diet that is low in fat, devoid of processed sugar and starches, and high in fiber, is essential for stabilizing blood sugar. Fiber-filled foods like beans, peas, and whole-grain and oat bran products will help balance your blood sugar. Avoid table sugar, as well as sugar in processed and prepared foods. Get your sweet fix from fruits.

Supplements/Herbs. In addition to a multivitamin-mineral supplement, consider taking supplemental chromium picolinate or brewer's yeast, which may help lower blood sugar naturally—but after you have discussed it with your provider.

235

Mind-Body Methods. Because yoga eases stress, it may help lower blood sugar.

Hands-On Healing. Massage and reflexology can minimize stress. For those whith advanced diabetes, acupuncture can reduce the pain and nausea associated with nerve damage.

Diabetes: Are You at Risk?

To find out if you are in danger of developing diabetes, take this quiz developed by the American Diabetes Association. Write in the points next to each statement below that is true for you. If a statement is untrue, write in a zero. Then total your score.

I am overweight (consult doctor if you're not sure).	Yes 5	____
I am under 65 years of age and get little or no exercise during a usual day.	Yes 5	____
I am between 45 and 65 years old.	Yes 5	____
I am 65 years old or older.	Yes 9	____
I am a woman who has had a baby weighing more than 9 pounds at birth.	Yes 1	____
I have a sister or brother with diabetes.	Yes 1	____
I have a parent with diabetes.	Yes 1	____
	Total	____

If you scored three to nine points, you are at low risk for having diabetes now but your risk may increase in the future.

If you scored ten or more points, you are at high risk for having diabetes. Only a doctor can determine if you have diabetes. See a doctor soon and find out for sure.

Heart Disease

What It Is

Heart disease is just one of many conditions that affect the heart and cardiovascular system. The form of heart disease most familiar to us is a heart attack, an event typically caused by blockage in arteries that prevents blood and oxygen from traveling through the heart. Angina (chest pain), atherosclerosis (hardened arteries), and congestive heart failure are other forms. Heart disease is more common in black women than doctors once believed, especially women over 50. It is caused by a combination of factors including poor diet, high cholesterol, lack of exercise, smoking, obesity, genetics, and stress. Because people with diabetes or hypertension are at increased risk, sisters are doubly in danger of developing heart disease. Emotional problems such as depression or anger can raise the risk. The symptoms are often silent; even heart attack symptoms mimic those of other benign conditions, and they may be different in women. Those symptoms include:

- Pressure, tightness, or pain in the chest
- Shortness of breath
- Extreme fatigue
- Nausea
- Dizziness
- Sweating or clamminess and cool skin
- Indigestion

Because recent research indicates that doctors may miss heart attack signs in black women and not refer us for further testing as often as they refer whites and men, it's important to listen to your body. If something doesn't feel right, it probably isn't, so don't hesitate to go to the hospital if you think you might be having a heart attack, and insist on proper care.

How to Detect It

Doctors may use a variety of tests to determine whether someone has had a heart attack or may be at risk of having one. A standard test is catheterization, in which a doctor inserts a catheter or tube in the arteries to assess their health. Additional tests include an electrocardiogram, which measures the heart's muscle activity and can detect a heart attack that does not have symptoms.

Prevention and Complementary Care

Lifestyle. Regular exercise strengthens the heart and encourages weight loss. One study showed that women who walked briskly for 3 hours per week cut their risk of heart attack by about a third. Get regular physical exams and stay on top of treatment for diabetes or hypertension.

Nutrition. A low-fat, high-fiber diet containing whole grains (brown rice, oatmeal) reduces heart disease risk. Soy has also been proven beneficial to the heart.

Supplements/Herbs. In addition to a multivitamin-mineral, you may benefit from extra folic acid; talk to your provider about dosages. Supplemental garlic, coenzyme Q10, fiber and fish oil also benefit the heart.

Mind-Body Methods. Deep breathing and meditation relieve stress. Because research has proven that negative emotions such as depression and hostility can affect the heart, therapy or support groups may help you prolong life.

Hands-On Healing. Massage and reflexology may benefit the heart.

Resources

American Diabetes Association, National Service Center, 1660 Duke Street, Alexandria, VA 22314; (800) ADA-DISC.

American Heart Association, 7270 Greenville Avenue, Dallas, TX 75235; (800) 242-8721, or see the yellow pages for a local office.

National Diabetes Information Clearinghouse, Box NDIC, 9000 Rockville Pike, Bethesda, MA 20892.

National Heart Lung and Blood Institute, PO Box 30105, Bethesda, MA 20842-0105; (800) 575-WELL.

Diabetes, by David M. Nathan, MD, with John F. Lauerman (Times Books).

Her Healthy Heart: A Woman's Guide to Preventing and Reversing Heart Disease Naturally, by Linda Ojeda, PhD (Hunter House).

The Healthy Heart Formula, by Frank Barry, MD, with Bridget Swinney, MS, RD (Chronimed Publishing).

Natural Remedies for a Healthy Heart, by David Heber, MD, PhD (Avery Publishing).

The Other Diabetes: Living and Eating Well with Type 2 Diabetes, by Elizabeth Hiser (Morrow).

Heart Health for Black Women: A Natural Approach to Healing and Preventing Heart Disease, by Dr. Beverly Yates (Marlowe and Company).

Chapter 14

~

Emotional Healing: Stress, Depression, Phobias

NATURAL WOMAN: EVE ROBINSON

Since the days when she didn't like going to crowded amusement parks as a child, Eve Robinson always felt a little anxious around a lot of people. But it wasn't until she was in her late thirties that her anxiety became a problem. First there was the time she began to feel like she was choking while driving on the freeway and had to pull over, vowing never to get on the highway again. Then months later, her heart started racing after she boarded a plane. Certain that she was going to die, Eve begged the flight attendant to let her off. Slowly she grew more fearful and her world grew smaller until she could no longer even leave her house. Eve's panicky feelings became her prison. Though she couldn't pinpoint the fear, she remembers its intensity: "You think when you leave the door, you're going to die."

From home, she contacted a therapist, who helped her gradually find her way back. In therapy, Eve learned, in addition to having been sensitive as a child, the trauma of watching her father die suddenly when she was twenty might have triggered the development of her panic attacks. To cope, she learned how to reduce her anxiety by writing in a journal, deep breathing, swimming for exercise, and drinking herbal teas. She uses positive self-talk to nip panicky feelings in the bud. "When I get anxious . . . I tell myself everything is going to be okay," she says. "I try to breathe." Taking lavender baths and drinking kava kava tea also help.

Though she hasn't gotten back on a plane, Eve has resumed most normal activities and even launched her own nonprofit organization, the Sankofa Holistic Healing Institute in Oakland, California. In addition to offering resources such as a healing journal for people with anxiety disorders, the institute held its second annual conference in February 2000, bringing together individuals and medical experts to discuss alternatives to coping with anxiety. The success of the institute and the focus on helping others aid Eve in her own healing. "I try to stay focused on helping other people." She adds: "I feel like I'm really doing good work and making a difference."

Behind the façade of black women's super strength and spiritually based power lie a host of emotional ills and pain, including low self-esteem, anxiety, anger, phobias, and depression. Though, according to all the stereotypes, we are supposed to be domineering, independent, aggressive superwomen, we face the same—and in some cases more—psychological stresses and concerns as anyone, yet we are not allowed to express them. As the thinking goes, if we survived slavery, what have we got to complain about?

These myths and misconceptions mask our very real need for emotional healing. Black women have a 50 percent higher rate of clinical depression, the most common form of depressive illness, than white women. Approximately one in three sisters are grappling with the fallout of sexual abuse. Others suffer from panic attacks and anxiety disorders, as well as more severe forms of mental illness such as schizophrenia. In many cases, because of a lack of awareness, shame, and bias in the medical system, our mental health problems go underdiagnosed and undertreated. This causes many of us to suffer silently and needlessly until emotional problems overwhelm us, or worse, we simply get used to them. The lack of an outlet for emotional pain pushes many sisters to addictions of all kinds—to food, alcohol, cigarette smoking, or drugs.

But black women are survivors. One major source of our emotional strength is our faith and spirituality. Another is our growing number of sister support groups and circles. Through these outlets, we've learned there is no shame in laying our burdens down. Slowly we are also entering the offices of black mental health practitioners as well, taking off that mask of invulnerability to find that our true strength lies in telling the truth and healing from within.

Natural Healing Is Our History

Unlike many people in the West, indigenous Africans do not ignore or stigmatize emotional pain or the need for healing. In fact, according to Sobonfu E. Somé, author of *Welcoming Spirit Home: Ancient African Teachings to Celebrate Children and Community,* Africans often address these challenges through rituals. Expressing grief, anger, and other forms of emotional pain is not only acceptable, but is given importance through a ritual that invokes community as well as the ancestors and spirit. Describing a friend's ritual to heal old psychological wounds, Somé writes, ". . . she went to the shrine and spoke from her heart, in a non-blaming way, how hurt she has been by her own wounds, by lack of attention to her inner child, and by her feelings of worthlessness." She continues, "She let herself experience her rage and anger. At first she felt timid and small, but as the community supported her in her pain she found the strength and courage to continue." Through this ritual, which ended with a symbolic cleansing of the woman's wounds in water, she was able to not only release her pain but ask for support and receive it from her community.

Our West African ancestors encouraged the expression of psychological needs as well as the continual practice of healing through rituals. With the support of community, nature, and spirit, an individual or individuals could enter into rituals that allowed them to release pain that would otherwise cause them illness. Admitting to emotional difficulties and asking for help is not something for "crazy white people"—it is in our African tradition.

Black Women's Blues: Stress and the Sources of Our Emotional "Dis-ease"

As black women, we experience emotional stress every day but we're not always conscious of where our stress originates and how it affects our emotional well-being. Some sources of our stress and emotional "dis-ease" are societal—poverty, racism, sexism, violence, crime, poor health care, inadequate housing, single parenting, over-whelming family and community demands. Others—isolation and loneliness—are internal. The legacy of slavery still casts a shadow over many sisters' lives, denying us basic political and economic power, and a secure sense of self-worth. Being at the bottom of the socioeconomic ladder while struggling to achieve, keep our families intact, and uplift the race can be staggeringly stressful. Yet we seldom stop to acknowledge these challenges, take care of our needs, and seek relief.

Stress in and of itself may not cause mental illness but it con-tributes to it. Though heredity and biological factors play a role in many mental disorders, ongoing stress triggers the development of them. The stress of having been abandoned as a child may make us susceptible to depression as adults. The stress and trauma of having suffered child abuse or sexual abuse may set the stage for an anxiety disorder. As black women, we have numerous sources of stress; un-derstanding your stress will help you cope with—and prevent—mental health challenges.

Mental Illness

Health experts now know that mental illnesses such as depression and panic disorder are not character flaws but common conditions with physiological as well as psychological causes. These conditions may be difficult to diagnose but they are all treatable.

Depressive Illness

The term "depression" encompasses several conditions that are characterized by a persistent sad mood. The two major forms of clinical depression are (1) unipolar, or major depression, and (2) bipolar, also called manic depression.

Major Depression. Feeling sad from time to time is normal as is feeling depressed over a major loss or life change such as divorce. But when that sadness settles in like a cloud for several weeks to several months and does not go away, you may have major depression. Women are more likely to be depressed for reasons that may be hormonal but are not completely understood. Some mental health experts believe that certain people are predisposed to depression either genetically, biologically, or by traumatic events such as separation from a parent during childhood or sexual abuse. We then are more susceptible to becoming depressed when difficulties arise. (In some cases, depression is triggered by a physical condition such as diabetes or thyroid disease.) The first depressive episode usually occurs before age 20. You may be clinically depressed if you have four or more of the following symptoms for longer than two weeks:

- Persistent sad, anxious, or empty mood
- Lack interest or pleasure in activities you once enjoyed
- Changes in appetite; weight loss or gain
- Lack of sleep or oversleeping
- Restlessness, irritability
- Fatigue, lack of energy
- Feelings of worthlessness, guilt
- Inability to think clearly, concentrate, and make decisions
- Persistent physical problems such as headaches, chronic pain, constipation
- Suicidal thoughts or attempt at suicide

Understanding and acknowledging these symptoms is critical for black women: We are more likely to be depressed than white women, but because of a lack of awareness and persistent stigmas about mental illness in the black community, we may suffer silently and needlessly. Research on black women suggests that we may experience more of certain symptoms than others such as difficulty concentrating, sleep changes, changes in appetite, or physical health problems but not associate them with depression. The high rate of overeating and obesity among sisters may also mask emotional pain.

Being depressed is nothing to be ashamed of but it is something to take very seriously. If you think you are depressed, and especially if you've had thoughts of killing yourself, talk to a mental health professional. Psychologists, psychiatrists, psychotherapists, social workers, and spiritual counselors are trained to help you seek the best treatment. Your treatment will likely consist of therapy and possibly medication for at least six to twelve weeks. Those with mild or moderate depression may rely on therapy alone. Several complementary remedies are effective in helping cope with depression (see p. 251).

Manic Depression. Like major depression, manic depression is characterized by periods of deep sadness, but these lows alternate with periods of hyperactivity and elation, or mania. A person with manic depression or bipolar disorder may not know she is depressed because during manic phases, she feels invincible. During these periods, a manic depressive might spend recklessly or engage in risky sexual behavior. The causes of manic depression include some combination of genetics, biology, or chemical imbalance, and emotional problems such as trauma or chronic stress. The depressive part of bipolar disorder is much like major depression; the manic part may include these symptoms:

- Feelings of elation, euphoria
- Inflated self-esteem or grandiosity
- Loss of need for sleep
- Compulsive talking
- Racing thoughts; thinking up of many ideas simultaneously

- Distraction
- Increased activity in social, work, school, or sex life; compulsive planning
- Risky behavior such as overspending or increased sexual activity

Reviewing this list, and asking those who know you well to review it with you, is important because blacks with bipolar disorder are more likely to be misdiagnosed with other conditions such as schizophrenia. If you suspect you have manic depression, see your health care provider, who may refer you to a psychiatrist or other mental health practitioner. Consider bringing a family member or friend for support. Manic depression is not curable but you can manage it with a combination of therapy, medication, and complementary therapies. Research shows blacks with manic depression are also more likely to receive less treatment, so persist until you find what works for you.

Minor Depression or Dysthymia. Another less commonly known form of depression is dysthymia. A person with dysthymia simply feels sad all or most of the time. Though a person with mild depression may be able to function at work or in school, her life is dominated by feelings of anxiety and guilt. If you are irritable, pessimistic, and self-critical much of the time, you may have dysthymia. The causes are not well understood; they may include an inherited tendency or a chemical imbalance. The classic symptoms include:

- Poor appetite or overeating
- Lack of sleep or oversleeping
- Low energy
- Low self-esteem
- Inability to concentrate or make decisions
- Inability to experience emotions such as grief, joy or pleasure normally
- Hopelessness

Black women must be especially careful of a condition such as mild depression since it can sneak up on you and begin to feel like a normal part of life. Though dysthymia is a mild depression, it can last for many years. Half of those diagnosed with dysthymia will suffer major depression. Treatment consists of therapy or medication or both. Complementary therapies may help as well.

Postpartum Depression. About one in ten new moms will experience sadness, irritability, and other depressive symptoms within the first few weeks after giving birth. Unlike mothers who have the "baby blues," women with postpartum depression experience a deep, lingering sadness as their predominant mood. In addition to the typical signs of depression, women may also have negative feelings about motherhood and even want to harm their child. On top of the depression, women may feel ashamed and guilty for having less than motherly feelings. Experts believe postpartum depression may be triggered by the dramatic change in hormones that occurs after pregnancy and exacerbated by the physical and emotional demands of motherhood. Women who have a history of depression and those who have manic depression are more at risk.

As with any form of mental illness, we must take signs of postpartum depression seriously and get help. It is quite normal to experience sadness even during a time when women are supposed to be happy. For your sake and your child's, don't grin and bear it. Talk to your provider about using therapy, medication, or complementary remedies to heal.

Seasonal Affective Disorder (SAD). Triggered by shifts in daylight hours during seasonal change, seasonal affective disorder is a form of depression that can disrupt people's lives for five months or more. If you are susceptible to SAD, you may experience a depressed mood, anxiety, fatigue, sleepiness, and cravings for carbohydrates or starchy foods in the fall and winter months. You may feel too lethargic to go about your normal activities. At winter's end, your mood and energy level return to normal. SAD is more common in women and those who live in Northern states, where there is less light. SAD may be caused by an imbalance in certain hormones that affect mood or by a faulty body clock. Even though SAD tends to subside on its own, because it can last as long as October through April, if you suspect you have SAD, you should take steps to alleviate it. Light therapy, or exposure to artificial light from specially designed bulbs or light boxes, is an effective treatment. Some medications and alternative therapies such as meditation and cognitive therapy may also help.

Anxiety Disorders

We all feel anxious at times, but when worry and fear dominate our thoughts or prevent us from living our lives fully, we may have an anxiety disorder. These conditions, including panic attacks and post-traumatic stress disorder, are the most common mental health challenges nationwide.

Phobias. Fear of flying or being in enclosed spaces such as an elevator are familiar examples of phobias. These intense, irrational fears of animals, places, objects, or situations often cause physical symptoms such as sweating, rapid heartbeat, shortness of breath, trembling, nausea, or a panic attack. Specific types of phobias include agoraphobia, or the excessive fear of being in public places, and social phobia, the fear of embarrassment or failure during a public activity such as public speaking or attending a party. The cause of a phobia may stem from an inherited tendency if it runs in your family, a chemical imbalance in the brain, and/or a stressful or traumatic experience. Whatever the cause, phobias can be controlled through therapy, with medication, and with complementary techniques.

Panic Disorder. The fear that you are dying or having a heart attack without cause or actual danger is a sign of a panic attack. Other symptoms include sweating, rapid heartbeat, chest pain, shortness of breath, hyperventilation, dizziness, trembling, chills, choking, and nausea. An attack may come on suddenly with no apparent cause. During an attack, you may also feel an overwhelming sense of doom and unreality. After an attack, you may fear having another and avoid situations and places associated with the first attack. Having frequent panic attacks, four or more in one month, means you have panic disorder. Like phobias, panic attacks may be caused by a combination of genetics, biology, and stressful experience such as divorce or separation. Getting treatment for these problems early is key: Research has shown that blacks with panic disorder have higher rates of emergency room visits and hospitalizations than whites with panic disorder. Treatment may consist of therapy, medication, and/or alternative techniques such as cognitive therapy.

Generalized Anxiety Disorder (GAD). Having ever-present and uncontrollable feelings of fear or nervousness that last for six months or longer is known as generalized anxiety disorder. It is "generalized" because there is no specific source of anxiety but an overall sense of doom. This condition may cause physical symptoms such as sweating, rapid heartbeat, headaches, insomnia, and fatigue. Though GAD is not as severe as other forms of anxiety disorder, feeling tense without relief all or most of the time can rob you of a normal life. Treatment may consist of therapy, medication, and/or complementary techniques such as acupressure, deep breathing, and imagery.

Obsessive Compulsive Disorder (OCD). Repeated hand washing and checking of locked doors are familiar examples of this condition. OCD has two components: obsessive, uncontrollable thoughts about an anxiety such as contracting germs; and compulsive behavior to calm the anxiety such as returning home to check and recheck the locks. A person with OCD may develop compulsive rituals, such as rearranging objects, which can last for hours but never truly resolve anxiety. A similar disorder known as trichotillomania, or compulsive hair pulling, may be related to OCD. Though the behavior of a person with OCD simply seems odd, it can interfere with normal living and even lead to thoughts of suicide in many cases. Treatment may consist of therapy, medication, and/or complementary techniques.

Post-Traumatic Stress Disorder. "Shell shock" in war veterans is a common example of this condition, but survivors of many other types of trauma, including sexual abuse and natural disaster, may experience post-traumatic stress. To be diagnosed with PTSD, you must have either recurring, distressing memories of the event; recurring nightmares or daydreams about the event; flashbacks or hallucinations as if the event were happening again; intense fear of people, places, or things that remind you of the event. You may also experience intense and alternating feelings of vulnerability and rage. Traumatic events may also include child abuse, molestation, rape, battering, or crime. The symptoms may last for months or years, making it difficult for the sufferer to enjoy normal activities and function. Treatment may consist of therapy, medication, and/or complementary techniques.

Prevention and Complementary Care

Natural healing techniques can help you create emotional balance. Because mental illnesses are not just "in your head," but caused by a combination of mind-and-body factors, they benefit most from mind-and-body healing. You may need to experiment with a variety of strategies to see what works for you. (If you take medication, talk to your provider before using complementary techniques.)

Lifestyle. Regular exercise boosts energy and oxygen to the brain. It has been shown to help prevent and alleviate depression. It also reduces stress and anxiety. Consistency is key: do what you enjoy— walking, aerobic—four to five days a week.

Nutrition. Eating a balanced natural diet high in complex carbohydrates such as beans, whole-grain breads, and pastas can help alleviate depression by boosting the brain's mood chemical, serotonin. Avoid sugar, caffeine, and alcohol, which all negatively affect mood.

Supplements/Herbs. Take a multivitamin-mineral supplement to prevent nutritional deficiencies that might undermine emotional balance. The herbs St. John's wort, gingko biloba, and kava kava may all help to alleviate mild depression. Homeopathic remedies may also be beneficial.

Mind-Body Methods. Relaxation techniques such as meditation and progressive muscle relaxation all help lower stress. Deep breathing brings more oxygen to the brain, which benefits mood. A form of talk therapy known as cognitive-behavioral therapy is effective in treating anxiety disorders. Journaling, support groups, and prayer are additional stress busters.

Hands-On Healing. Certain forms of massage are designed to help people heal from emotional trauma.

Resources

Association of Black Psychologists, PO Box 55999, Washington, DC 20040-5999.

Black Psychiatrists of America, 41 Central Park West, Suite 10C, New York, NY 10023.

The National Association of Black Social Workers, 8436 West Mc-Nichols Avenue, Detroit, MI 48221.

National Foundation for Depressive Illness, Inc., PO Box 2257, New York, NY 10116; (800) 248-4344.

National Mental Health Association, 1021 Prince Street, 3rd Floor, Alexandria, VA 22314-2971; (800) 969-6642.

National Institute of Mental Health, Information, Resources and Inquiries Branch, Parklawn Building, Room 7C-02, 5600 Fishers Lane, Rockville, MD 20857; (888) 8-ANXIETY.

Can I Get a Witness: Black Women & Depression, by Julia Boyd (NAL-Dutton).

What Mama Couldn't Tell Us About Love, by Brenda Wade, PhD, and Brenda Lane Richardson (HarperCollins).

Willow Weep for Me: A Black Woman's Journey through Depression, by Meri Nana-Ama Danquah (One World/Ballantine).

Overcoming Panic Disorder: A Woman's Guide, by Lorna Weinstock, MSW, and Eleanor Gilman (NTC/Contemporary).

Your Mental Health, by Allen Frances, MD, and Michael B. First, MD (Scribner).

Index

INDEX

anti-inflammatory, 56
antinuclear antibody test (ANA), 204
antioxidants, 63–64, 66, 68–69, 216
antiseptics, 74, 85
anxiety, 133, 134, 241–242, 247–248
  disorders, 249–251
aphrodisiacs, 74
appetite, changes, 245–247
application of herbs, 77–85
Apresazide, 203
Apresoline, 203
armpit, 218
aromatic herbs, 78
arousal, sexual, 135
arrhythmia, treatment of, 64
art therapy, 102
arterial embolization, 161
arteries, 230, 237–238
arthritis, 43–44, 79, 124, 133
artificial menopause, 189
asanas, yoga, 13
ashtanga, yoga, 13
aspirin, 56, 76
assessment, self *see* tools, self-assesment
asthma, 23, 44–45, 64, 133
astragalus membranaceus, 80
asymmetry, of breasts, 218
at-home
  acupressure, 125–126
  birth, 163–164, 177–178
atherosclerosis, 237
athletes, 114–115
atoms, unstable, 68
attitude, positive, 105, 185
Ausar Auset Society, 151
auto-antibodies, 203–204
awareness, body, 4–8
Ayensu, Edward S., 73
Ayurvedic diet, 43

babies, bottle-fed, 179
"baby blues," 248
back pain, 157
bacteria, 143
bacterial vaginosis, 146
balance, 4, 61, 119
balanced foods, 40–41
balm in Gilead, 93–94
barriers to pregnancy, 170–172
basal body thermometer, 169
baths, 125
beans, 37, 39–40, 58, 65, 143
before pregnancy, 166–170
Beloved, 92
benefits
  of breastfeeding, 179
  of menopause, 186
  of psychotherapy, 100
benign tumors, 152–153, 218–219
beta-carotene, 58, 62, 67, 69
"Big C" *see* cancer
biofeedback, 99
biopsy, 143, 205, 221

bios (life), 40
biotin, 59
bipolar depression, 245–247
birth, 163–181
  at-home, 163–164
  underwater, 178
birth control pills, 56
birthing rooms and centers, 177–178
Black Adoption Consortium, 174
Black Adoption Placement and Research
    Center, 174
black cohosh, 75
bleeding
  excessive, 137–138, 141, 153, 157
  heavy, 137–138
bloating, 66, 126, 133, 134
blockage of arteries, 237
blood, 45, 58, 115, 116, 133
  clotting, 59, 60, 67
  purification with herbs, 74
  tests, 8, 47, 204
  thinners, 76
blood pressure, 61
  sudden dropping of, 47
blood proteins *see* antibodies
blood sugar, 45, 58, 61, 64, 234
  reactions, 44–45
blood-type, diet, 41–42
Blues, the, 244
blurred vision, 234
body wraps, 125–126
bone marrow, 59, 224
"bone setters," 115–116
bones, 61, 115, 195–196
  degeneration, *see also* osteoporosis
  development, 58–59
  fractures, 204
boron, 60
botanical medicines *see* herbs
bottle-fed babies, 179
brain, 58, 99, 140
bran, 39–40, 65
bread, 39, 45, 65, 232
breast
  cancer, 147–148, 211, 213, 222–223
  changes, 147–148
  clinical exam, 7–8, 219
  pain, 134
  self-exam (BSE), 217–219
  swelling, 134
  tenderness, 133
breastfeeding, 179–180
breasts, fibrocystic, 147–148
breath
  awareness, 96–97
  shortness of, 237
breath work, 96–97
breathing
  alternate nostril, 97
  conscious-connected, 102
  deep, 90
  exercise, yoga, 13
  and meditation, 96

INDEX

Index

INDEX

Index

INDEX

INDEX

INDEX

Index